Rozela Xhemnica

Application and clinical significance of biological age in dentistry

AF138576

Rozela Xhemnica

Application and clinical significance of biological age in dentistry

LAP LAMBERT Academic Publishing

Impressum / Imprint

Bibliografische Information der Deutschen Nationalbibliothek: Die Deutsche Nationalbibliothek verzeichnet diese Publikation in der Deutschen Nationalbibliografie; detaillierte bibliografische Daten sind im Internet über http://dnb.d-nb.de abrufbar.
Alle in diesem Buch genannten Marken und Produktnamen unterliegen warenzeichen-, marken- oder patentrechtlichem Schutz bzw. sind Warenzeichen oder eingetragene Warenzeichen der jeweiligen Inhaber. Die Wiedergabe von Marken, Produktnamen, Gebrauchsnamen, Handelsnamen, Warenbezeichnungen u.s.w. in diesem Werk berechtigt auch ohne besondere Kennzeichnung nicht zu der Annahme, dass solche Namen im Sinne der Warenzeichen- und Markenschutzgesetzgebung als frei zu betrachten wären und daher von jedermann benutzt werden dürften.

Bibliographic information published by the Deutsche Nationalbibliothek: The Deutsche Nationalbibliothek lists this publication in the Deutsche Nationalbibliografie; detailed bibliographic data are available in the Internet at http://dnb.d-nb.de.
Any brand names and product names mentioned in this book are subject to trademark, brand or patent protection and are trademarks or registered trademarks of their respective holders. The use of brand names, product names, common names, trade names, product descriptions etc. even without a particular marking in this work is in no way to be construed to mean that such names may be regarded as unrestricted in respect of trademark and brand protection legislation and could thus be used by anyone.

Coverbild / Cover image: www.ingimage.com

Verlag / Publisher:
LAP LAMBERT Academic Publishing
ist ein Imprint der / is a trademark of
OmniScriptum GmbH & Co. KG
Heinrich-Böcking-Str. 6-8, 66121 Saarbrücken, Deutschland / Germany
Email: info@lap-publishing.com

Herstellung: siehe letzte Seite /
Printed at: see last page
ISBN: 978-3-659-79710-1

Zugl. / Approved by: Albania, Medical University of Tirana, Faculty of Dental Medicine, 2015

Copyright © 2015 OmniScriptum GmbH & Co. KG
Alle Rechte vorbehalten. / All rights reserved. Saarbrücken 2015

Ph.D. ROZELA XHEMNICA (RROÇO)

MONOGRAPH

**APPLICATION AND CLINICAL SIGNIFICANCE OF
BIOLOGICAL AGE IN DAILY CLINICAL PRACTICE**

2015

Recognition

I want to express my gratitude to the scientific leaders of the study Prof. Xhina Mulo, for the launch and completion of this project, for her help and valuable suggestions throughout the research work.

I thank my colleagues at the University Dental Clinic (FMD), and my family for their support and encouragement throughout this period.

I sincerely appreciate the cooperation of all patients and their parents involved in this study, who agreed to participate without personal gain, but seeking progress of science.

FORWARD

Growth or postnatal development starts from birth and ends when adult maturity is reached. The process of maturity is achieved when growth and development of an individual have reached a point at which it is possible to perform any appropriate action and function or maintain certain stability. The status of development of a child is not correctly assessed in most cases based on the chronological age alone, but by biological age. There are three physiological parameters that determine the life developmental events and the biological cycle of growth: Endochondral ossification (stages of bone morphology at hand-wrist level), dental age (teeth formation and eruption), and secondary sexual signs (secondary sexual characteristics). Biological age is regularly used in pediatrics, and is widely used in orthodontic treatment planning to assess if the patient is approaching, has reached or passed the peak of pubertal growth. Determination of the biological age is very important to achieve, because it has a larger spectrum in the medical field, besides dentistry. Knowledge of the maturity stage that a child has reached can assist in the evaluation of his progress through the anticipated developmental events. Such information is clinically important because it helps the interdisciplinary medical teams to assess deviations from the norm for patients with different types of short stature, with endocrine disorders and / or metabolic diseases etc. Its usefulness lies in identifying syndromes and forensics. Many types of orthopedic treatment in general medicine also require accurate assessment of patient maturity status.

CONTENTS:

1. INTRODUCTION

Malocclusion of teeth is a disorder that affects the teeth-jaw-face apparatus and its treatment is a primary responsibility of the physician orthodontist. In daily practice the successful treatment of dental and skeletal anomalies depends on the timing of the intervention and mechanotherapy used. (2,3). The study of the changes that occur in the facial complex helps clinicians to identify and diagnose any existing anomaly, in order to ensure optimal treatment for the patient. It is therefore essential for the dentist to be aware of how the face changes and where and when such changes occur. Such knowledge helps to modify the processes of growth. Clinicians are concerned as to the immediate results of treatment, as well as long-term stability and benefits of treatment, because changes in the face and dentition continue throughout life. At certain stages of development these changes are drastic and easily observable. While at other times the changes are more subtle, but of equal importance. i.e. when normal individuals between the ages of 25 and 45 were studied, significant changes in dental-facial complex were observed. These changes include greater prominence of the nose and more emphasis of dental agglomeration. The status of development of a child is not correctly assessed in most cases based on the chronological age alone, but by biological age. There are three physiological parameters that determine the life developmental events and the biological cycle of growth: Endochondral ossification (stages of bone morphology at hand-wrist level), dental age (teeth formation and eruption), and secondary sexual signs (secondary sexual characteristics). (1,5) Due to obvious individual variations that determine somatic maturity at any chronological age, age of growth presents often a measure a more measure to determine the development of a child compared to chronological age, especially when a diagnosis needs to be established for a patient with an altered pace of growth and also a treatment plan in terms of interceptive orthodontic or Dental-facial corrections. When assessing a child's progress towards maturity, generally doctors make a comparison between his stages comparing standard results obtained from samples in a population of the same age. (6;45).

In this field are used indicative standards such length in orthostatic position, weight, skeletal development, secondary sexual characters and dental development. This way it is possible to evaluate if the child's maturity is in the early stages, intermediate or delayed compared to his peers. (9). The practice and the clinical experience of many foreign authors has shown that if the before treatment of abnormalities, especially the skeletal ones, the timing of intervention is not accurate, the result will be either complete failure or extension of treatment in time! The concept of growth and development.

All dentists should have *a sufficient knowledge of craniofacial growth and development.* The study of not only the dentition development, but the entire dental-facial complex, *is a professional duty in order to i favorably intervene in the facial growth.*

Why study growth?
1. To identify abnormal pathological growth
2. To diagnose any significant deviation from normal norms
3. To understand the changes in occlusion and jaw during growth
4. To plan treatment
5. To determine the appropriate effects of treatment.

Most orthodontic treatment occurs in growing children. Orthodontists should be aware of:
1. Effects of treatment after growing stops
2. To increase the impact of growth in the progress and outcome of treatment
3. How growth can help or impede orthodontic treatment.

If orthodontist does not have a clear and quantitative assessment of growth at the beginning of treatment, it will be impossible to assess the progress of treatment later!
Terms growth and development are closely related, but they are not synonymous.
Growth is an anatomical phenomenon that includes increasing in size and number.
Development is a physical phenomenon that includes growth, organization, complexity or specialization.Postnatal human growth includes the physical, mental, psychological and moral components.
Human physical growth is a sequence of events that converts 1 single cell in an individual of complex nature. Humans spend 30% of their life growing. (14,21).
This long period causes situational factors to influence the biological system that is growing. Growth is a combination between circumstantial and hereditary factors.
Growth is an increase and change.(23).
No definition can explain the complexity of growth. Although most of the growth cycle is completed around 20 years of age, some tissues such as hair and nails continue to grow throughout life.

There are three periods of growth: *infancy, childhood, adolescence.*
- Infancy includes the first year of postnatal life.
- Childhood is divided into: a) early phase (1 to 6 years), b) secondary phase (6 to 10 years), c) the late phase (10 to 12 or 13 years).
- Adolescence-going from 14 to 20 years in men and 13 to 18 in women.

These are general guidelines and do not include the extremes of variations, which may occur in the postnatal growth.

There are different types of growth:

1. Changes in size: changes in size while growing are easily recognized and measured in many ways: weight (mass); height, length and width (thickness); perimeter, area and volume.

2. Positional change: tissues and organs can migrate from one area to another during growth. An example is the erupted tooth.

3. Proportional change: parts of the body vary in relation to each other during growth. Infant head in proportion to the body is much bigger than the head of an adult.

Cephalocaudal growth gradient - Scarnmons: There is a growth axis that extends from the head towards the feet.

In fetal life, about the third month of intrauterine development, the head comprises about 50% of the total length of the body and the cranium is relatively wide compared to the face. Trunk and extremities are rudimentary. At birth, the head occupies 39% of the total body length, while the foot-1/3 of the total body length. In an adult the head occupies about 12% of the total body length, while the feet-1.2 total of body length. Therefore, with the growing process trunk and extremities grow faster than the head and face.

Diagram presenting the cephalocaudal growth gradient (27)

4. Functional change: tissues and organs are subject to change in functional abilities during the growth process. The purpose of growth is the mature functioning of each tissue of the body.

5. Maturing change: body growth as a whole is moving in the direction of achieving a period of stability and the adult status.

6. Compositional change: growth includes changes in the composition of certain body parts. Eye pigmentation changes and body water content is down from 90% in the fetus, to approximately 65% in adults.

7. Changes in time and sequence: continued growth lasts from conception till death, but for many reasons the growth rate varies for different parts of the body.

Certain growing stages can be identified:

a. Prenatal growth is characterized by the rapid increase in the number of cells and the fast pace of growth.

b. Postnatal growth is characterized by reduced growth rates and tissue growing maturity.

c. Maturity is a period of stability during which the body reaches its maximum function and processes of growth limited to maintaining a balance between the process of cell loss and gain.

d. Old age is a period during which functional activity and growth processes are lowered.

8. Changes in the growth speed: the curve of growth speed. Various authors have divided this phase into three periods (98):

-The p*eriod of Childhood,* is characterized by a high degree of initial growth which falls rapidly.

- *Juvenile period* is characterized by a relatively slow growth, lowering into early adolescence.

-*Period of Adolescence* is characterized by a noticeable increase in the rate of growth reaching its peak during puberty, followed by a decline in the rate of growth until the end of growing cycle and with the advent of adult age.

For women the period of adolescence begins by age 10, reaching a peak growth at age 12 and ending at age 17. For boys in adolescence usually starts two years later. However there are different variations of the individuals of both sexes. The speed of the increase in pubertal peak is 8.5 cm per year for girls (standard deviation SD = 1 cm) and 10 cm per year for boys (standard deviation SD = 1 cm).

This way the boys are taller than girls because the juvenile period lasts longer and they develop at greater speed at the peak period of pubertal growth. (44) (52) (53)

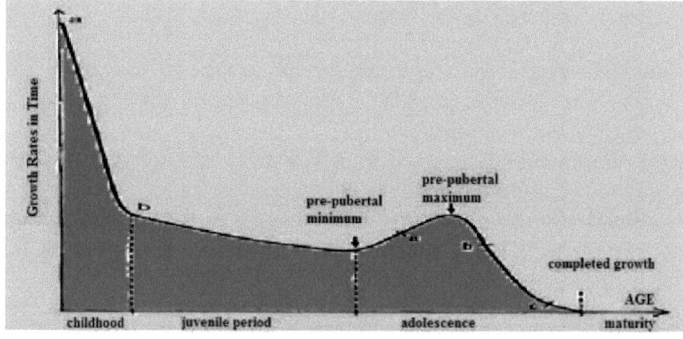

Speed growth curve

The major factors influencing growth are divided into:
I) Endogenous factors: genetic, functional, neurotrophic, hormonal.
II) Exogenous factors: environmental, nutritional, affective, socio-economic,
etc ..

1. Genetic factor. Basic control of growth in magnitude and time is localized in
the genes.
The potential for growth is genetic. The actual outcome depends on the growth
potential interaction between genetic and circumstantial influences.
Studies of twins have shown that the size, body shape and type of growth are all
under genetic control more than what is circumstantial.
Brodie has published some interesting studies in the 40-s, presenting the
hypothesis of a close genetic control in facial morphology (cartilage and sutures
are controlled by genetics). According to this theory cranium growth is
predetermined and is not subject to external influences and so it is relatively simple
to predict growth. (51). Genetic factors also play an important role in the growth
differentials male-female. A more pronounced development in girls compared to
boys in terms of maturity is attributed to delayed action of the male Y
chromosome. By delaying growth the Y chromosome allows men to grow for a
longer period of time than women and consequently the overall growth is greater.
Individuals with XXY type chromosome (Klinefelter's syndrome) have very long
feet and have a kind of growth similar to men. Individuals with Turner's syndrome
have only one X chromosome and have a similar growth pattern as women.
Individuals with the XYY chromosome have too long of a constitution which
support the hypothesis that the Y chromosome has a delayed effect on growth.
2. Functional Factor. The importance of functional factors is widely demonstrated
and more clearly in cases of aglossia, temporo-mandibular ankylosis. The essence
is the functional matrix hypothesis by *Moss*.
3. Neurotrophic factor. According to this theory neuronal activity controls
muscular activity and growth. Neuronal control of skeletal growth is defined by the
term "neurotropism". From a theoretical point of view it is likely a direct
neurotrophic effect on osteogenesis, but has not been demonstrated experimentally.
(54). Neurotropism can intervene indirectly affecting and influencing the soft
tissue growth, which in turn can control and modify the growth and skeletal
morphology (hypothesis of *Moss* on functional matrix). Currently it is not possible
to distinguish the neurotrophic effects on bone from the muscular one.
4. Hormonal factor. Growth hormone (GH or HGH), also known as somatropinne
or somatotropin hormone, is a peptide produced by the pituitary gland
(hypophysis).

During adolescence, the plasma levels of the growth hormone significantly increase, stimulating the growth in stature, promoting nitrogen retention in the body and favoring oxidation of lipid deposits. All these effects are mediated by IGF-1 (somatomedin or an insulin-like growth factor), a strongly anabolic hormone produced by the liver in response to somatropinne. (46). Once the period of adolescence has passed the levels of GH decreases but nevertheless the body continues to produce the hormone. Somatotropin hormone in adult age plays an important regulatory role in various metabolic processes. (62). GH plasma varies in values from 1 to 5 mg / ml points to 10 mg / ml in case of stress or after a hard exercise. Residual GH secretion was pulsatile reaching higher frequency and wider spread in the early hours of night sleep. Discovered in 1912 by *Evans*, GH has been subject of studies in order to assess the therapeutic effects and possible side effects.(95). A deficit in GH in children compromises body growth (pituitary dwarfism), the development of genital organs and somatic tracts, simultaneously causing an increased adipose accumulation in the abdominal region. If lack of GH occurs in adults, there is reduction of muscle mass and the simultaneous growth of adipose mass, metabolic alterations other signs, as well as increased and decreased bone fragility and lowering in exercise tolerance.

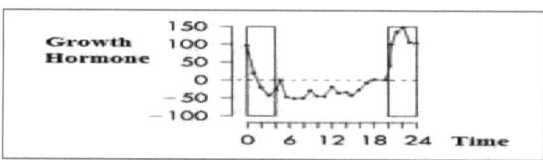
GH (growth hormone)

Also, thyroid hormones, thyroxine and triiodothyronine hormones, both stimulate the overall metabolism and are important in the growth of bones, teeth and brain. Lack of iodine reduces the production of these hormones. Thyroids secretion decreases from birth to adolescence and then explodes during pubertal growth. It is agreed that the pituitary and thyroid hormones play a small direct role in the explosive growth of a teenager. The first changes in adolescence are caused by the secretion of androgens and gonadal hormones. Androgens are produced by the suprarenal cortex, which is controlled by Adrenocorticotropic hormone (ACTH), produced by the pituitary gland. (74). No significant difference in the amount of ACTH occurs during adolescence, so we thought that perhaps a mechanism for inhibiting androgen production occurs during adolescence to allow secretion of androgens.

Androgens play a major role during the teenage growth in both sexes. Gonadotrophic pituitary hormone stimulates the production of testosterone in men and estrogen and progesterone in women. Testosterone and adrenal androgen both stimulate the growth of muscle, bone, red blood cells and provide secondary sexual characteristics in males. Ovarian secretions have less overall influence in the growing process and in females the androgen production by adrenal glands is primarily responsible for the growth in teen years. Ovarian secretion controls secondary sexual changes, including alterations of the body.

5. Nutritional factor: continuous hyper-nutrition has a positive effect on growth and the maturation of endochondral ossification; otherwise mal-absorption and malnutrition are associated with a slowdown in growth and bone maturation. (8;30). Malnutrition includes deficiency in calories and nutritional elements needed. Hunger strikes change body composition, protein are consumed but not accumulated, so the body cell mass is reduced. (58). Fat is consumed. Extracellular fluid increases. 9 amino acids are essential for growth. The absence of any of them results in growth disorders. Calcium, phosphorus, magnesium, manganese and fluoride are essential for the growth of bone and teeth. Iron is needed for the production of hemoglobin.Vitamins are also essential for normal growth. Vitamin A controls the activities of both osteoblasts and osteoclasts. Defects in bone growth occur in the absence of vitamin A. Vitamin B2 has considerable influence on growth. Vitamin C is necessary for bone and cognitive tissue growth. Vitamin D is required for normal bone growth. (109). Animals that followed a diet in calories stopped growing. When added enough calories in the diet, they began to grow again. This kind of adaptation of the body to different diets also occurs in humans. (90) The growth of teeth has precedence over bone growth and bones grow faster than soft tissues, such as muscles.

6. Exogenous factor, such as the action of **orthodontic apparatus** on mandibular structures, is known as an important modifier of their growth, at the age of child growth and development. (93)

7. The socio-economic factor contains in itself several components such as level of education and income of the parents, their profession, values and individual behavior or attitudes. These factors exert significant influence on the growth of the child. (7;60;61).

The trend in the new century

There is considerable evidence that children today are growing faster than in the past. The trend is probably a result of better nutrition and a balanced diet. Other reasons are low morbidity and improved health care. Although children are growing quickly their growing cycle also ends faster. Early in the 20th century, boys reach the final height at age 25; nowadays this age is 20 years old.

The new standards should be regularly determined in relation to the sustainability of the parameters in this century, conditioned by improving the nutrition and health verified in the 20th century that have influenced significantly the degree of maturity and the final weight.

The views and contemporary studies by different authors about the accelerated growth in modern times.
It has long been said that females reach puberty sooner. A studio of Max Planc, Institute for Demographic Research in Rostock, Germany (47), managed to demonstrate that the age of sexual maturation is also changing in boys, while in girls the age of sexual maturity is very easy to identify, marked by the arrival of menstrual cycle (menarche), so by the first menstrual flow. Some scientists see the early arrival of the menstrual cycle as a social devastation, because the phase of childhood is shortened and the sexual activity among girls increases. This way is increased the risk for pregnancies and sexually transmitted diseases. (48;26;43).

In boys the signs are not so clear, so scientists calculate the difference of chronological age from the age of sexual maturation male by analyzing data on mortality of boys. (25) When the production of male hormones reaches its maximum level the probability of death increases significantly. British experts call this *accident hump* (shore of the accident). (86). In real life precisely because of this hormonal storm young boys are more likely to take action, they are more active and often it is the momentum of such rash and furious actions that can cause incidents. Period of mortality in males who have reached adulthood broadly coincides with the peak of the male hormone production. (87).

Accident hump is common in all societies and according to experts coincides with puberty stage in which reproductive capacity is reached. (88). So by analyzing the peak of mortality, German researchers have determined that the pubertal peak is accelerated in comparison with the past, specifically it approached 2 and a half months every 10 years, starting from 1700

If calculations are made based on that, 18 years today means you have to have been 22 years old in 1800.
An explanation of this acceleration of sexual maturity in females as well as males:
According to experts this is the consequence of a number of environmental and nutritional factors. In urban areas of India the menarche age in girls was shown to be 12.6 years, as of Agawal data, which is similar to Menarche age in the developed world. (89;28). Although, large-scale data on the end of menarche age in rural areas in India are lacking, there is a general observation that the age of menarche is later, about 15-16 years in rural girls who are relatively weak and malnourished. In countries such as China and Senegal for which multiple data are available, the average age of menarche in rural areas is still high 16.1 years. (29).

Considered together all these data highlight the crucial role of socio-economic and nutritional factors, at the time of puberty. (30). Also, activities involving intense physical exercise which require a lot of energy at the age of puberty, have a negative impact in the development of the individual. In Western Europe where data are available for about the past 200 years the age of the menarche has changed from 17 years to 12.8 years. (31;32;55).

Mechanisms for the period of puberty
Curious researchers have tried to find the reasons for the phenomenon of the start of the menstrual cycle at an earlier age and have come to some conclusions. Improved nutrition and body mass, seems to be the most important contributors to early sexual maturity. (33) The authors have shown that a critical amount of fat mass is necessary for the onset of puberty and this is confirmed by many others. (90;57).

Weight is a measure widely used, but also an unsatisfactory indicator of somatic maturity. An increase in weight can be a result of growth, but also an increase in fat and the amount of water in the body. (34) In contrast, an adequate increase in length may be associated with weight gain, if at the same time there is a decrease in fat. (8) Overweight has an impact on sexual maturation. Many girls mature faster as a result of obesity. This aspect is very important to assess because the infantile obesity is increasing. (64;68).

Infantile obesity in the world: Infant obesity is a serious problem in many countries. Brazil has an incidence of 35% compared with 24% of obese (overweight) children in Italy. Many countries such as France have recorded a progressive increase of weight in children from 1963 to 2000. In America children with weight problems are growing and they reach about 70%. (83).

Intense psychological stress (as in time of war) is known to significantly delay the onset of the menarche, as suggested by data collected from Bosnia and Croatia. (35;36). Finally, chemicals such as Dichlorodiphenyltrichloroethane (DDT) have been shown to be in high amounts in children who enter puberty early. Time of exposure to these chemicals may affect the timing of puberty and may explain the phenomenon of early puberty in children adopted from developing countries.(37). Growth problems can be divided into two large groups of ***primitive and secondary*** problems. Primitive problems influence growth from pre-natal life, while the secondary problems appear on the post-natal age. Evidencing the difference between primitive and secondary problems is necessary for the diagnosis, treatment and prognosis because they vary significantly. In most cases primitive growth problems lead to a reduction in the age of adult stature. Secondary growth concerns can be treated with good results and the normal length can be reached frequently in adult age, if the appropriate treatment starts at an early age. (1)

Primitive growth problems	Secondary growth problems
• Skeletal dysplasia.	• Malnutrition
• Congenital metabolic defects	• Systemic and metabolic diseases
• Chromosomal aberrations	• Dwarfism
• Short stature born cases	• Conditional delayed growth

Factors that provoke post-natal growth problems

Different standards or the methods used for assessing growth by biological age.

Biometric parameters of assessing growth

Control of growth through anthropometric measuring starts in prenatal life, through ultrasound and continues after birth. The normality anthropometric measures are judged by reference to tables or graphics standards, generally in the form of curves of growth. (22) .The numbers we get by measuring the weight and length of a large number of children of the same age take into account gender, ethnicity and environmental factors.

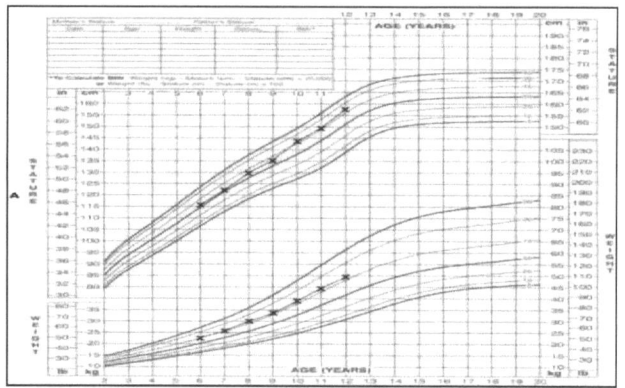

The speed of growth for females

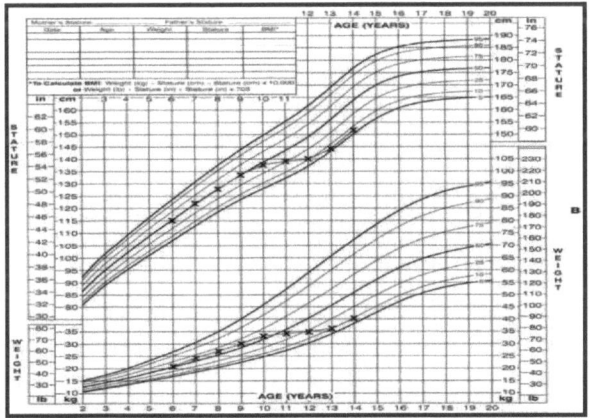

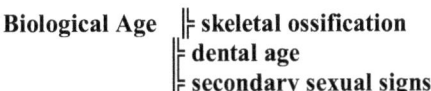
The speed of growth for males

Evaluation of weight and length which is done every 6 months identifies the speed of growth and repeatedly shows if there is an acceleration or deceleration of growth.(24). The status of development of a child cannot be evaluated in most cases using the chronological age alone. There are three physiological parameters that determine the development of life events, is the biological cycle of growth. (59)

Biological Age ╠ **skeletal ossification**
        ╠ **dental age**
        ╠ **secondary sexual signs**

Assessment of biological age based on skeletal age
According to foreign authors the link between the ages of bones with the child's stages of growth is very accurate. Skeletal age assessment is based on signs of maturing stage within the skeletal system. Different areas of the skeleton are used to determine skeletal age, foot, knee, elbow, cervical vertebrae, and shoulders. Bone ossification of the hand and wrist (stages of mineralization carpus, metacarpus, phalanges) is normally the evaluation standard for skeletal development. (98). Bone age assessment is a procedure often performed in pediatric radiology. Radiological examination demonstrates the skeletal development of the left hand, bone age is estimated and then it is compared with chronological age.(42;11).

15

This examination is used universally because of its simplicity, minimal radiation exposure and validity of multiple assessment ossification areas which help in assessing maturity and also increase the reliability of the analysis. A radiograph of the hand and the wrist provides a view of 30 small bones, which have a predictable Endochondral ossification order . This gives an accurate picture of the status of the child's skeletal development, therefore is considered *"accurate biological clock"*. (18;19;20).

Reminders and a bit of history
Skeletal maturity is a continuous process up to a certain age and refers to the degree of development of bone ossification. During growth, each bone undergoes through a series of changes that can be seen in radiological tests. When *Roentgen* demonstrated his new discovery of X-ray (Ro) in 1895, *Roland* introduced (1986) the notion of radiographic superposition to compare the size and shape of the growing bones as an indicator of the level of growth. In 1900 *Pryar* and *Crampton* began their experiment on the indicators of maturity on consecutive X-rays of the wrist and growing hand. *Hellman* published his observations on the ossification of epiphyseal cartilage of the hand, in 1929. *Wingate Eodal* started a longitudinal study in 1931 by taking a series of regular Ro of hand and wrist in children growing up in Cleveland, Ohio area. *Prof. Eodal* died in 1938 after the publication of the raw data of the study. After his death, the study was continued by *Grenlich-Pyle* who published the book *"A radiographic atlas of the skeletal development of the hand and wrist"* published in 1950 and revised in 1959-1972. *Fishman and Bjork*, in 1982, did a more complete interpretation of the respective Ro. Indicators of skeletal maturity (IMS) containing developmental changes involved in the process of bone enlargement of epiphysis, diapophysis coverage, and diaphyseal-epiphyseal fusion. (103).

Other methods of determining skeletal age:
► In Japanese schools an indicator of the patient's skeletal maturity is endochondral ossification in the distal phalanx of the thumb. Diaphyseal-epiphyseal fusion of the distal phalanx of the thumb occurs maximally 1-3 years after the pubertal growth in the Japanese population. (9).
► Another method that was used by Todd was the determination of skeletal age by referring to the first, second and third hand fingers. To determine the validity of the method used the variability analysis of ANOVA was used. Todd tried to determine whether consideration of only one part (3 fingers) of an area of the body (hand-wrist) would be enough to determine the skeletal age with a precision similar to the case when we consider the whole hand-wrist area. The difference between the two methods regardless of sex and assessment time was only 2.1 months. As shown by ANOVA both methods have a great statistical difference.

However, for clinical purposes the three finger method can still provide relevant information and is comparable to the hand-wrist method. This method helps in clinical evaluations of the growth potential of the patient and simplifies timing and types of orthodontic treatments, as well as the appropriate time for surgery. (119)

▶ Several European schools use the vertebrae. The maturity of the first 7 vertebrae in the spinal column constitutes the cervical plug. Maturing changes can be observed from birth to full maturity (91;15;84;85).

Lamparski used cervical vertebrae and has found them as reliable and available as the hand-wrist areas to determine the skeletal age. He has developed a series of standards for the assessment of skeletal age for females and males. This method has the advantage of eliminating the additional X-ray tests, because the vertebrae are registered in lateral cephalometric radiography. (71;72;73). So they used the anatomical changes in Ro cephalometric cervical vertebrae (81). This method has two disadvantages:

1. Maturing indicators undergo small changes over time and is not easily visible as are those in the hand area.

2. An incorrect position of the neck makes the visualization of vertebra difficult. Relationship between vertebral maturation stages of the change in mandibular growth before puberty is not studied yet. As a result of the growth stages of cervical vertebrae are related to mandibular growth during puberty (4;16). So changes in the stages of cervical vertebrae can be used to determine the time of mandibular growth during puberty. Although perfected standards for determining skeletal age are only from 10-15 years old, this is a stage when orthodontic treatment is often performed and determination of skeletal age becomes more important. (17;10).

Indicators of bone maturity (skeletal) in children and adolescents.

Most healthy children have a steady continuation of ossification of carpal and metacarpal bones and of phalanges which is a notable continuous process and is the same for both sexes. In general, the first bone area that shows in the X-rays of the hands and wrists, is the capitate bone and the last one to show is often the sesamoid bone of the visible parts of the thumb.(79;104) The first epiphyseal area to appears is that of distal radius, followed by those of the proximal phalanx, metacarpal bones, middle phalanx, distal phalanx and the end ulna. There are, however, two exceptions to this order; epiphysis of the distal phalanx of the thumb, usually displayed at the same time as the epiphysis of the metacarpal bone and the epiphysis of the middle phalanx of the fifth finger, which is usually the last to ossify. Given that the estimated value ossified centers varies and changes during growth, seeing in retrospect should primarily focus on centers that best reflect the age of the skeletal development during growth subjects. (69).

Assessment of biological age according to dental age.
Dental maturity and dental age constitute a method used to assess the biological age based radiology. ***Demirjan*** system is the system most widely used but other systems have developed with reference systems of the Nordic countries. (38). Maturity can be estimated by counting the teeth in the mouth after we have ensured that the child is in a period of active eruption. Demirjan system is very broad and is based on analyzes carried out in 4700 Franco-Canadian subjects. The system is based on the examination of the teeth 31-37 in a panoramic x-ray of the bottom left quadrant. (39;40;41). There may be large variations between chronological age and dental age. Various population and ethnic groups may represent different values and for this reason the differences between population under screening and the population we are referring to, should be taken into account i.e. adopted children, who may not know the exact date of birth and there are no accurate data on the population from which they have originated, makes it difficult to determine the exact chronological age of the child. Assessment of dental status is important in order to determine the prognosis of dental development and the connection with the biological maturity. Due to numerous variations in the formation of the tooth, it seems that the methods based on the stages of formation are more suitable to assess individual age than those based on other indicators of somatic development.(99). Stages of the calcification are used to determine the dental age. (63;75). Dental age determination is done based on dental mineralization stages of dental letters, where the stage of development of certain teeth seen by "Ro", is compared with a predetermined degree of maturity. This procedure is used during the temporary and mixed dentition and is not influenced by premature loss of baby teeth. (101;102).

9 respective stages of dental development
O- Dental germ shows no signs of calcification
A- Calcification of certain occlusal contact points without the fusion of different calcified areas
B- Fusion points mineralized; occlusal contours seen
C- Coronary amelogenesis is completed: the deposition of dentin starts
D- Conclusion of the formation of crown to glaze-cement merger
E- Radicular length is shorter than the coronary height
F- Radicular length is equal or greater than the coronary height
G- Completion of radicular formation; the apical foramen is still open
H- The apical foramen is closed; periodontal membrane around the root and the apex is even in width.

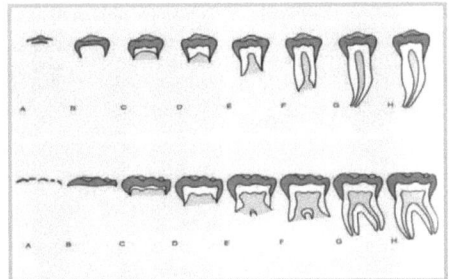
Dental mineralization stages of mono and multiradicular teeth

Assessment of biological age according to secondary sexual characteristics.
Sexual development occurs through several stages, which vary from individual to individual. Stage of development of secondary sexual characteristics, provides a physiological adolescence calendar, pertaining to the status of individual physical growth, so there is a high correlation between the ratio of sexual signs and pubertal peak. Adolescence in girls can be divided into 3 stages based on the extent of sexual development (76;65).

In **the First stage,** which occurs at the beginning of the curve, there is an immediate explosion of physical growth which is easily observed by parents and is as easily referred to the doctor.
The peak or the highest curve of physical growth is about 1 year after the start of stage I and coincides with **Second stage** of development of sexual characteristics, which become quite visible (development of breasts, the emergence of vegetation).
Third stage in girls occurs 1 year or1 year and a half after the second stage and is characterized by the start of menstruation.

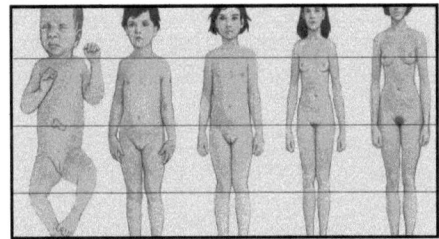
Developmental stages of sexual characteristics

The stages of sexual development in boys are more difficult to specify than girls. Puberty starts 2-3 years later and extends to a period of about 5 years compared to the 3 and a half year period of sexual development in girls.

In boys there are 4 stages of development associated with the growth curve of the body in adolescence:

Stage I: an initial sign of sexual maturation in boys is usually the weight gain. Guys that are starting to mature gain weight due to the production of estrogen.

In stage II: 1 year after the first stage, there is a pronounced growth in height while there is a relative reduction of weight.

Stage III: occurs 8-12 months after stage II and coincides with the peak of the rapid growth, is characterized by addition in height. At this time facial vegetation appears, muscular growth occurs, change of voice, as a result of deterioration of balance hormonal glands overproduction of fat. Also, a clear sign is the appearance of the characteristic face acne.

Stage IV: this stage occurs 15-24 months after the III-d stage and is difficult to ascertain. At this stage the pronounced growth in height ends and vegetation appears on the chin. For obvious reasons maturing indicators that require physical examination of sexual characters are not applicable in clinical orthodontics.

Also, in cases of non-referral by the mother, the discovery of such characteristics, as the increase in height, change of voice, etc., requires longitudinal chase. Therefore this method of determining the biological age cannot be considered as the primary method but it assists in determining the maturing status.

The importance of determining biological age in orthodontic treatment

The dentist should have a deep understanding of growth and physical development and should be able to contribute to the diagnosis of growth rates in young children. A normal growth is possible only if the child is healthy and takes from takes from the nutritional diet the factors needed for optimal growth and development. Recognition of skeletal age is very important in the diagnosis and treatment of children with variable growth, in order to discover if there is a delay in growth coupled with the associated variations of skeletal maturity. (70).

2. PURPOSE OF STUDY

Conducting methods to determine biological age is very important for every clinician who deals with children that are growing and developing. Knowledge of the maturity stage that a child has reached, assist in the evaluation of his progress through the anticipated developmental events. Such information is clinically important because it helps the interdisciplinary medical teams to evaluate patients with different types of short stature, with endocrine disorders and / or metabolic diseases. Its usefulness lies in identifying syndromes in forensics medicine as well. Many types of orthopedic treatment in general medicine also require accurate assessment of patient's maturing status. It is important to determine the age of the patient because now in orthodontic practice in 50-60% of cases, the chronological age does not match the real skeletal development of the patient, while ***Biological age*** is being recognized and valued.

The greatest success in orthodontic therapy is possible at the time of biggest changes. This means that the period just before and during the growth spurt is regarded as an advantageous period for the application of various types of orthodontic treatment (49). So in orthodontic treatment planning, it is relevant to predict if the growth spurt has just begun or if it has been completed. This way, a positive result is achieved by using the mechano-therapy in the treatment Dental-facial deformities and a clear prognosis is evidenced at the start of treatment.

The main objectives of this paper are:
- ➢ 1. Assessment of dental maturity, based on the method panoramic X-Ray through the Demirjan method.
- ➢ 2. Assessment of skeletal maturity based on the radiographic appearance of the calcified structures of the hand and wrist, as well as the respective ultrasound.
- ➢ 3. Identification of inconsistencies and discrepancies between the actual chronological age and the biological one(skeletal, dental and sexual)
- ➢ 4. The use of orthodontic mechano-therapy based on biological age in skeletal cases.

3. MATERIAL AND METHOD

Method and selection of subjects

Our study was conducted in a total of 160 patients aged 7-15 years, 90 girls and 70 boys, at the University Dental Clinic and a private clinic. All patients had dental and skeletal anomalies (the choice of selection was ours). The period of study was 2009- 2012. For each group predetermined criteria defined in advance, was followed, based on the work by foreign authors who have conducted similar studies and clinical investigations.

Inclusion criteria for patients in the study:

-*First*: this study included patients who had dental and skeletal anomalies, without any history of previous orthodontic treatment.

-*Second:* this study included healthy subjects who did not suffer from any primary disease such as endocrine or nutritional disorders, since these disorders affect the development of the subject.

-*Third:* this study included patients that were clinically free from any prolonged or chronic disease, so they had normal growth and development.

Methods used in the study:
Subjective examination

This examination is useful to determine the patient's good health. It is useful to have an idea of the height and weight of the patient, they should be measured occasionally and these data should be placed in a growth chart (Somatogram). During the *subjective* examination, in the interview conducted with the patient and especially during the interview with the parent, one of the most important moments the determining of the general status of the patient based on age, weight and height.During the subjective examination we assess the biological age through the establishment of: skeletal age, dental age and sexual maturity stages.

Some of the questions relating to secondary sexual characteristics that we ask the mother and the female patients are about the start or not of the menstrual cycle, breast development, the appearance of vegetation and what is readily observed by parents and doctor, the immediate physical growth spurt.

Regarding male patients, questions that doctors ask in order to ascertain the stage of sexual development are about weight gain, height increase, facial vegetation,, change of voice as a result of the disruption of the hormonal balance, the presence of face acne as a result of overproduction of glandular fat.

Extra-oral objective examination includes:

▶ During this examination we observe the brachyfacial and dolichocephalic facial type.

In the case of dolichocephalic facial type there is a formation of elongated cranium characterized by a reduced biparietal diameter (distance from one ear to the other) and by an increase in the anteroposterior diameter (fronto-occipital diameter), then the distance from the point of nose contact with the forehead to the point of exit of the occipitals'. Brachycephalic facial type, means a more rounded head, where length and width are nearly equal. The ratio of these two measurement ranges from 0.82 -1.

▶ The next step of the objective extra-oral examination is to assess the lips and see whether they classify as competent or incompetent. Labial competence is achieved by closing the lips in silenced mode without any muscle strain. The lower lip is supported in the third lower vestibular surface of the upper incisive. Labial incompetence is examined by closure of the lips in the position of tranquility with strained muscles which may depend on:

- Skeletal discrepancy of the sagittal or vertical type

- Serious case of dentoalveolar discrepancies etc.

▶ Assessment of floors of the face, to see the normal existence of equality between 3 floors superior, middle and inferior among them.

▶ Profile Assessment form: concave, convex or harmonic (right).

Facial profile is determined by observing the anteroposterior view.

Soft tissue profile is reflected on the skeletal profile.

To begin the examination the child sits at straight position gazing out to some distal point. Three points of the face are identified: the tip of the nose, the upper lip base and chin. The lines that connect these points form an angle that makes the face appear convex, straight or concave.

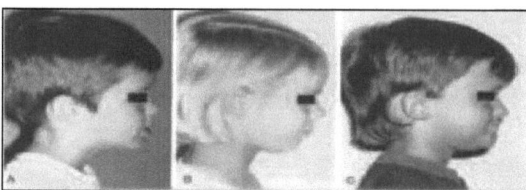

A. Class II is characterized by a well-balanced profile of anteroposterior dimension. This profile is created by drawing imaginary lines that join the tip of the nose, upper lip (maxilla) and the tip of the chin (mandible). This line should be slightly convex. B. Class II is characterized by a completely convex profile. C. Class III is characterized by an anteroposterior concave profile.

Intraoral objective examination includes:
► Soft tissues, oral hygiene and periodontal condition involving oropharynx and tonsil
► Hard dental tissues
► Closing and orthodontic reports
► Dentition type (mixed or permanent)
► Frenulum
During the ***functional examination*** the entire masticator system was analyzed, and so we evaluated:
► The correlation between the position of stillness and central occlusion in order to identify whether the present functional abnormality is functional or skeletal
► Movements of the temporomandibular articulation and the possibility of touching, through the presence of pain in palpation, crepitations or non-synchronization of the two ATMs during the opening and closing the mouth
► Type of swallowing: normal or atypical swallow
► Type of respiration: nasal or oral
► Type of phonation

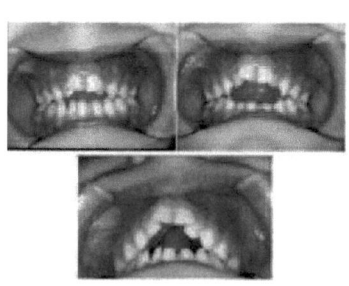

Atypical ingestion

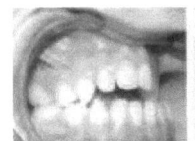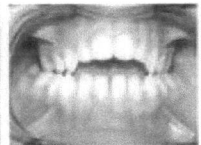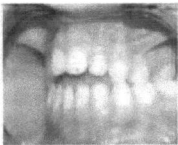

The anomaly created by oral breathing

▶Assessment of muscular activity: if the muscles have mobility and normal muscle tonification.

In the sagittal plane the occlusal ratio was assessed by determining the correct grade of the angle for the posterior area (molar classes), as well as for the anterior (canine classes).

In the vertical plane the open bite and overbite (open bite and deep) were assessed.

In the transversal plane the presence or otherwise the absence of cross bite, bite scissors, mono or bilateral and compliance of the median line, were determined.

In additional analyzes we used the panoramic graph to determine the dental age and Ro 'hand and wrist to determine the exact skeletal age.

▶Panoramic radiograph provides information about the growth and development of dental elements and bone structures. The number, location, dimension and shape as the crown, as well as the roots are determined. Also, dental follicles of developing teeth are examined.

▶ While the Ro' of hand consists in determining the skeletal age, that serves us to determine growth potential.

> **Determination of dental age**

In the panoramic graph a quad (left or right) in the lower jaw (not in the upper jaw, as the teeth sides up superimpose each other in panoramic Ro) is analyzed. We determined stages of mineralization of each tooth (mono or multi-radicular), which are assigned the relevant points in the table.

The amount of points for the 7 corresponding teeth is transported to another table, to be converted into dental age for both genders (male, female).

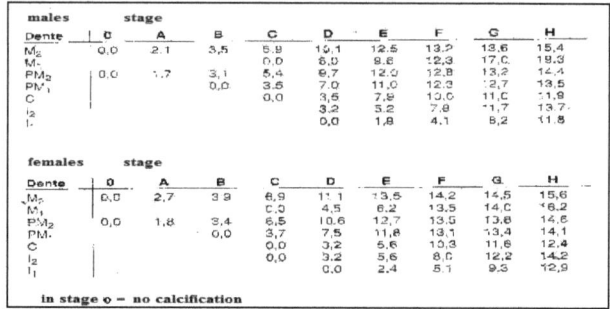

Respective points based on dental mineralization stages.

age	points		age	points		age	points		age	points	
A	M	F	A	M	F	A	M	F	A	M	F

Definition of dental age by accumulated points

> ### Determination of skeletal age.

In the clinical study and our work, we use the skeletal deciphering by Bjork, since that method is very simple, feasible by all and more reliable and secure.

Decoding in 9 stages by Bjork Regulation
Stage 1 (PP2)
Epiphysis of the proximal phalanx of the index finger represents a width equal to that of diaphysis (approximately 3 years before pubertal peak).

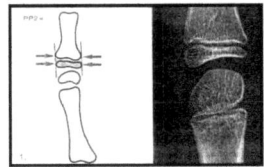
Stage 1

Stage 2 (MP3)
Epiphysis of the central phalanx of the middle finger presents the same width as that of diaphysis.

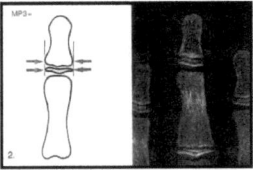
Stage 2

Stage 3 (Pisi+ H1+ R)
- *Stage Pisi* – Clear evidence of ossification of the Pisiform bone
- *Stage H1* – beginning of the ossification of Uncinato bone
- *Stage R* - Epiphysis and diaphysis of radius have equal width

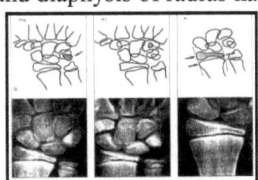
Stage 3

Stage 4 (S+ H2)
Before pubertal peak
- *Stage S* – The first mineralization of Sesamoid bone
- *Stage H2* – Complete ossification of Uncinato bone

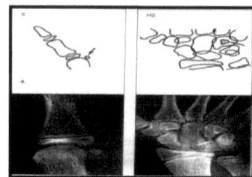

Stage 4

Stage 5 (MP3cap + PP1cap + Rcap)

Peak of pubertal growth. Epiphysis includes diaphysis in the shape of a cap.

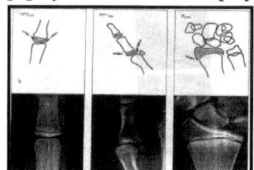

Stage 5

Stage 6 (DP3u)

The evident fusion of epiphysis and diaphysis corresponds to the distal phalanx of the middle finger. Growth peak is over.

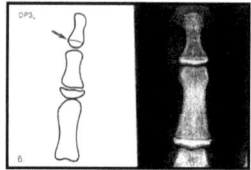

Stage 6

Stage 7 (PP3u)

The evident fusion of epiphysis and diaphysis in the proximal phalanx of the middle finger

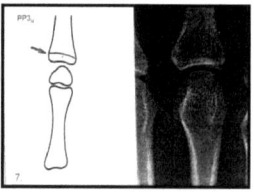

Stage 7

Stage 8 (MP3u)

The evident fusion of epiphysis and diaphysis in the central phalanx of the middle finger

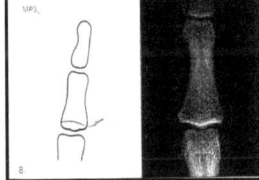

Stage 8

Stage 9 (Ru)

Complete fusion of the ossification of epiphysis and diaphysis of the radius..
At this stage, the ossification of all the bones in the hand is completed.

Skeletal growth ends

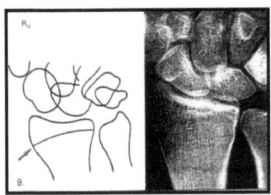

Stage 9

The chart shows the summarized presentation of the 9 stages Bjork Regulation and alignment with chronological age, in girls and boys.

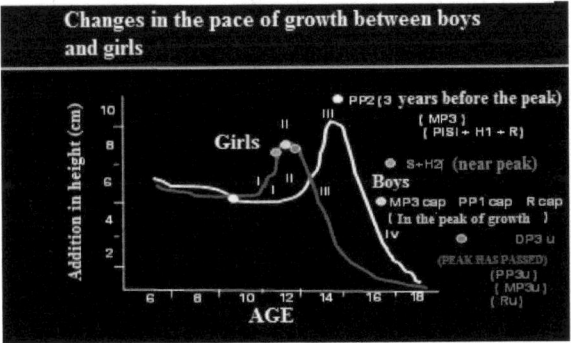

Graphic presentation of the stages of Bjork

In our study, a significant portion of the patients participating in the study also askedcephalometric-radiography.

Cephalometric analysis is used to specify the relationship of dento- alveolar and dento-dental bone structures in the anteroposterior and vertical direction. Lateral cephalometric analysis of the scalp is a common diagnostic tool that is used to determine the relationship between skeletal and dental structures. Cephalometry is recommended when there are obvious skeletal discrepancies and when a complete orthodontic treatment is being considered. Cephalometric analysis provides specific information about the contribution of each dental and skeletal component in malocclusion. Bone spots and skin spots can be seen; median point and lateral points. Points allow the determination of lines and planes needed for different cephalometric analysis. Lines and planes determined by the points that we discussed above and are parallel to the sagittal median plane. I n our study some patients asked for the ultrasound wave as an alternative method. **Hand Ultrasound**: In contrast to standard X-ray, ultrasound focuses on certain bones, from the beginning of ossification of their core.

4. STATISTICAL ANALYSIS

Continuous data were presented at their average value and standard deviation. Discrete data were presented in absolute value and percentage. Analysis between two groups with continuous data, were analyzed by using the Student test for two independent samples. Chi-Square test was used to identify differences for discrete data. Random links between variables were analyzed by multinomial regression analysis (when the dependent variable has more than two categories) and by binary logistic regression (the dependent variable was dichotomous, binary). For each variable was introduced OD (odds ratio) and confidence interval (CI) 95%. The Statistical analysis was conducted via statistical package SPPS 19.0. It was considered significant values of $p \leq 0.05$.

5. RESULTS

► **Patients according to dental and skeletal anomalies:**

Of 160 patients participating in the study, 120 (75%) were patients with skeletal abnormalities and 40 (25%) were patients with dental anomalies.

► **Patients according to dental and skeletal anomalies in connection with compliance / discrepancies:**

Compatibility	Skeletal anomalies (n=120) (%)	Dental anomalies (n=40) (%)	Total n=160 (%)
Discrepancy	81 (67.5)	20 (50.0)	101 (63.1)
Compliance	39 (32.5)	20 (50.0)	59 (36.9)

Patients according to dental and skeletal anomalies in connection with compliance / discrepancies

Using the Chi-Square test no statistically significant difference was evidenced between the groups (according to the type of anomalies) associated with dental compliance ($\chi2 = 1.19$, df = 1, p = 0.098), so the discrepancy is found in every phase and every type of abnormality.

► **Dental conformity and treatment starting time:**

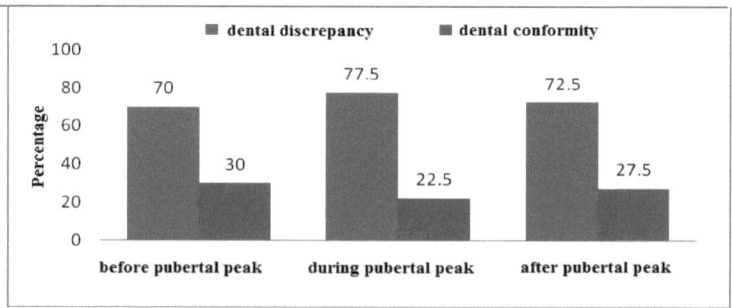

Dental conformity and treatment starting time

32

► **Time of treatment for skeletal anomalies**

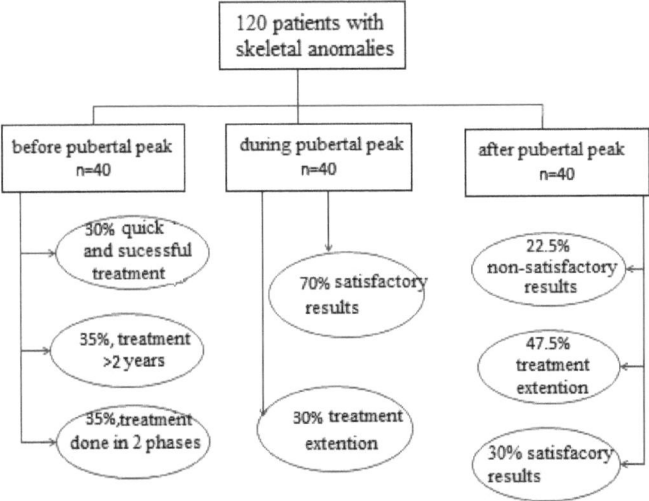

Through Chi-Square test a statistically significant difference was evident between groups (based on the time they start treatment) regarding the results of treatment. In the group that was treated at pubertal peak, satisfactory results were found in 70% of cases; much higher than those encountered in the group treated group after pubertal peak (30%) and the group before pubertal peak pubertal (30%) (p = 0.019). This indicates that if patients treated at peak pubertal have the best treatment results.

Results of treatment of skeletal abnormalities after pubertal peak

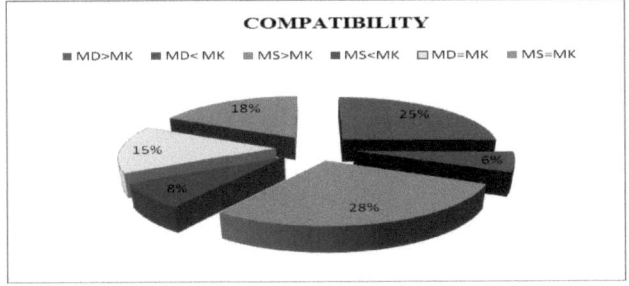

Compatibility of dental and skeletal age in relation to chronological age

► **Real age and the estimated one (dental and skeletal) for children at 7 years of age**

For children age 7, through the application of student test for two even pair samples results show that there is no difference between chronological age and the dental age in females (p = 0.057) and males (p = 0.113). Also, there is no difference between chronological and skeletal age of females (p = 0,118) and males (p = 0.134). Differences were absent in the total of this age group between the Chronological Age and the Dental Age (p = 0.134), as well as between the Chronological Age and the Skeletal Age (p = 0,073).

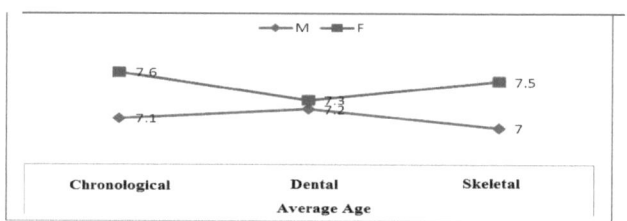

Real age and the estimated one (dental and skeletal) for 7 year old children

► **Real age and the estimated one (dental and skeletal) for 8 year old children**

For children age 8, through the application of student test for two even pair samples results show that there is significant difference between Chronological age and the Dental age in females (p=0.023) and males (p=0.015). Also, there is significant difference between chronological and skeletal age of females (p=0.017) and males (p=0.017). Differences were statistically significant in the total of this age group between the Chronological Age and the Dental Age (p=0,036), while there was no statistically significant difference in this age group between the Chronological Age and the Skeletal Age (p=0.057).

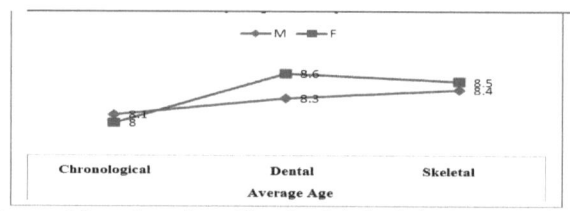

Real age and the estimated one (dental and skeletal) for 8 year old children

► **Real age and the estimated one (dental and skeletal) for 9 year old children**
For children age 9, through the application of student test for two even pair samples results show that there is significant difference between Chronological age and the Dental age in females (p=0.009) and males (p=0.011). Also, there is significant difference between chronological and skeletal age of females (p=0.047) but not for males (p=0.073). Differences were statistically significant in the total of this age group between the Chronological Age and the Dental Age (p=0,043), while there was no statistically significant difference in this age group between the Chronological Age and the Skeletal Age (p=0.057).

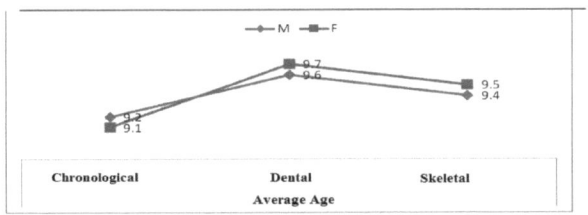

Real age and the estimated one (dental and skeletal) for 9 year old children

► **Real age and the estimated one (dental and skeletal) for 10 year old children**
For children age 10, through the application of student test for two even pair samples results show that there is significant difference between Chronological age and the Dental age in females (p=0.05) and males (p=0.013). Also, there is significant difference between chronological and skeletal age of females (p=0.014) and males (p=0.047). Differences were statistically significant in the total of this age group between the Chronological Age and the Dental Age (p=0,004), and also between Chronological Age and the Skeletal Age (p=0.013).

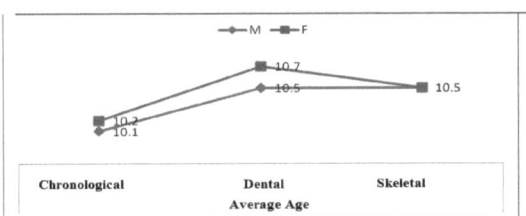

Real age and the estimated one (dental and skeletal) for 10 year old children

► **Real age and the estimated one (dental and skeletal) for 11 year old children:**

For children age 11, through the application of student test for two even pair samples results show that there is significant difference between Chronological age and the Dental age in females (p=0.001) and males (p=0.02). Also, there is significant difference between chronological and skeletal age of females (p=0.024), but not for males (p=0.07). Differences were statistically significant in the total of this age group between the Chronological Age and the Dental Age (p=0, 0014), but there was no significant difference between Chronological Age and the Skeletal Age (p=0.089), there was no statistically significant difference in this age group between Chronological Age and the Skeletal Age (p=0.057).

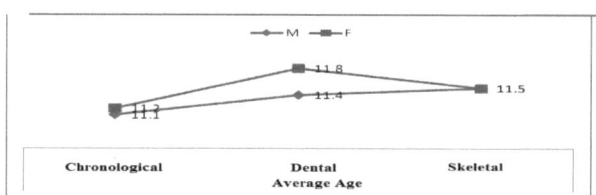

Real age and the estimated one (dental and skeletal) for 11 year old children

► **Real age and the estimated one (dental and skeletal) for 12 year old children**

For children age 12, through the application of student test for two even pair samples results show that there is significant difference between Chronological age and the Dental age in females (p=0.05) amd for males (p=0.013). Also, there is significant difference between chronological and skeletal age of females (p=0.003) and males (p=0.001). Differences were statistically significant in the total of this age group between the Chronological Age and the Dental Age (p=0,022), and also, between Chronological Age and the Skeletal Age (p=0.001).

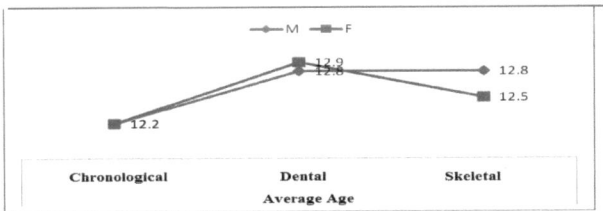
Real age and the estimated one (dental and skeletal) for 12 year old children

▶ **Real age and the estimated one (dental and skeletal) for 13 year old children**

For children age 13, through the application of student test for two even pair samples results show that there is significant difference between Chronological age and the Dental age in females (p=0.009) and in males (p=0.018). Also, there is significant difference between chronological and skeletal age of females (p=0.038) and males (p=0.001). Differences were statistically significant in the total of this age group between the Chronological Age and the Dental Age (p=0,001), and also, between Chronological Age and the Skeletal Age (p=0.001)

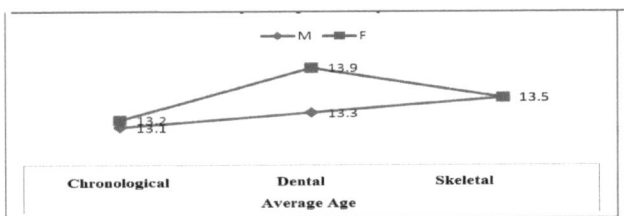
Real age and the estimated one (dental and skeletal) for 13 year old children

▶ **Real age and the estimated one (dental and skeletal) for 14 year old children**

For children age 14, through the application of student test for two even pair samples results show that there is significant difference between Chronological age and the Dental age in females (p=0.001) and in males (p=0.001). Also, there is significant difference between chronological and skeletal age of females (p=0.001) and males (p=0.002). Differences were statistically significant in the total of this age group between the Chronological Age and the Dental Age (p=0,005), and also, between Chronological Age and the Skeletal Age (p=0.004).

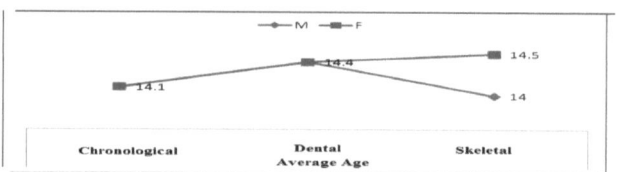

Real age and the estimated one (dental and skeletal) for 14 year old children

► **Real age and the estimated one (dental and skeletal) for 15 year old children**

For children age 15, through the application of student test for two even pair samples results show that there is significant difference between Chronological age and the Dental age in females($p=0.05$) and in males ($p=0.013$ Also, there is significant difference between chronological and skeletal age of females ($p=0.05$) and males ($p=0.013$). Differences were statistically significant in the total of this age group between the Chronological Age and the Dental Age ($p=0,005$), and also, between Chronological Age and the Skeletal Age ($p=0.036$).

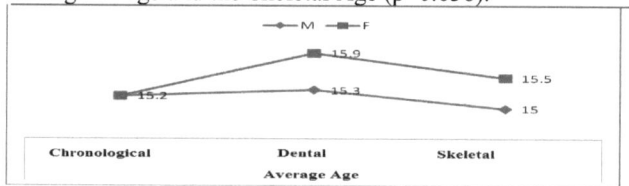

Real age and the estimated one (dental and skeletal) for 15 year old children

► **Real age and the estimated one (dental and skeletal) for children in total**

For the total of children, through the application of student test for two even pair samples, results show that there is significant difference between Chronological age and the Dental age in females ($p = 0:05$) and in males ($p = 0.013$). Also, there is significant difference between chronological and skeletal age of females ($p = 0:05$) and males ($p = 0.013$). Differences were statistically significant in the total of this age group between the Chronological Age and the Dental Age ($p = 0.007$), and also, between Chronological Age and the Skeletal Age ($p = 0.041$).

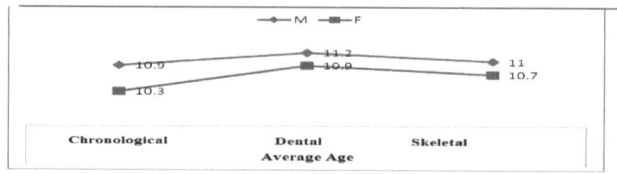

Real age and the estimated one (dental and skeletal) for children in total

38

6. CLINICAL CASES

Below we present some cases the patients that were examined. Through clinical examination and radiographs (panoramic, the wrist and hand, and they cephalometric), we assessed the dental and skeletal maturity.

1. Patient K.B. Anomaly: Second Class / dental and skeletal anomaly.
Patient 9 years and 10 months required treatment of upper teeth, which came out of the lips. Extra-oral examination shows a convex profile, an incompetent lip and anterior teeth that lie above the bottom edge.

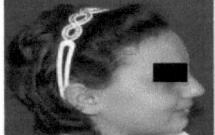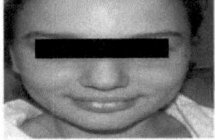

Extra-oral view

Intraoral view indicates the presence of over jet and II dental class.

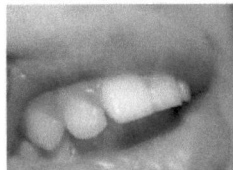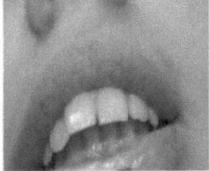

Intra-oral view

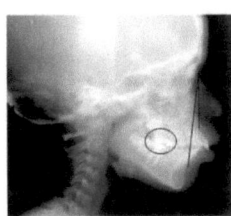 Cephalometric x-ray

Based on chronological age we were ready to start functional treatment immediately. While according to secondary sexual characteristics, patient's mother in in her reference shows that the girl has not yet entered the stage of maturity (before phase II). Also, the dental age of the patient was estimated at 8 years and 9 months (it was noted that premolars have erupted prematurely reducing dental calculating points), and the skeletal age was 8 years 11 months.

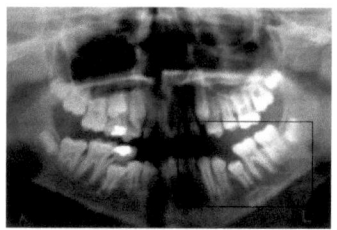 Panoramic X-Ray

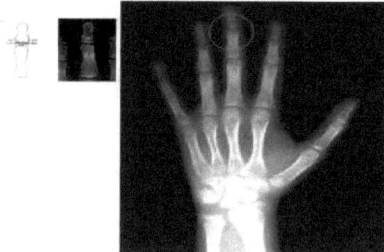 Hand and wrist X-Ray

Based on the following data:
Chronological Age: 9 years 10 months.
Skeletal age: 8 years 11 months.
Malocclusion: Class II / 1.

We decided to begin with functional orthopedic treatment at a later stage. But with the persistence of parents and especially of the patient who was concerned for her rabbit like appearance and wanted to fix quickly, we decided to start treatment, making clear that there would be 2 stages in treatment duration stretched for more than 2 years. In phase I was applied the activator for the advancement of dental mandibular and maxillary retrusion.

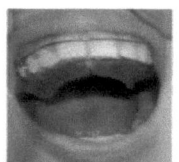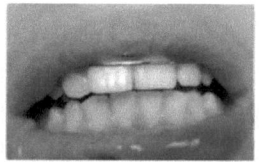

Stage I of treatment

After 2 years, Phase II of treatment began, wherein the apparatus intended to regulate the curve of spee to intrude the frontals and stimulate extrusion of the posterior teeth. As shown in the extra-oral view, the patient has visible signs of Acne on the face, which is one of the indicators that the girl has entered the stage of pubertal growth. Termination of treatment resulted in I-st dental and skeletal class.

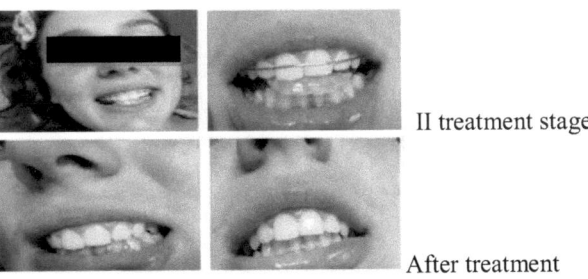

II treatment stage

After treatment

2. Patient S.V. Anomaly: Second/II dental and skeletal class
Patient is 15 years and 1month, required treatment of the upper teeth which were badly positioned. Extra-oral examination shows a convex profile, folded and retrusive lips and inferior low height

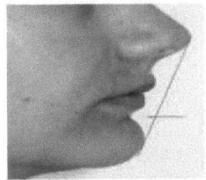

Extra-oral profile view

Intraoral view shows the presence of malocclusion II/2 class

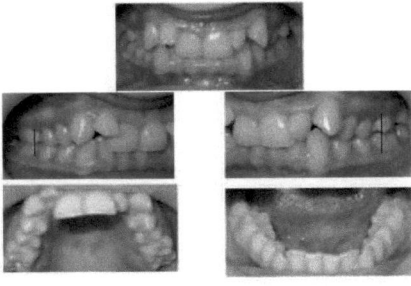

Intraoral view

41

The data from the anamnesis regarding the secondary sexual signs showed that the girl had passed the period of growth and skeletal development.

Age determination by use of panoramic X-Ray shows a dental age of over 16 years

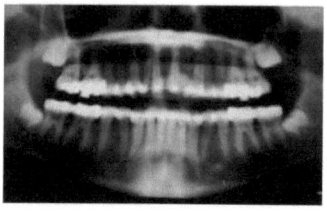

Panoramic X-Ray

While the determination of skeletal age by the hand and wrist radiographs indicates that the patient is in stage 8, so the patient has no more growing potential.

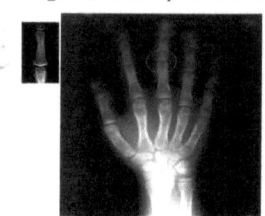

Hand X-Ray

By using the cephalometric method a diagnosis was determined: II skeletal class with mandibular retrusion and II / 2 dental classes.

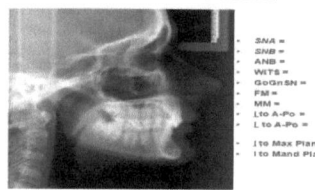

Cephalometric X-ray

Based on the following data:

Chronological age: 15 years 1 month.

Skeletal age: 16 years 4 months.

Because the patient does not have the growth potential, the treatment goal was to correct orthodontic dental grade and alignment of teeth in superior and inferior arcade. For this purpose 2 maxillary premolars were extracted.

42

Orthodontic treatment stages:
1) Extraction of the first superior premolars
2) The closure of premises and alignment of teeth in the superior dental arch.
3) Stripping in the inferior arch
4) Alignment and leveling of the arch
5) Leveling of Spee arc
6) Develop a stable occlusion

At first, after the extraction of 2 maxillary premolars, partial arches were used with the intention to increase anchorage and functional and stable occlusion and avoid the exaggerated vestibularization of the frontal incisive teeth and jiggling phenomenon. (Front-back movement of a tooth).

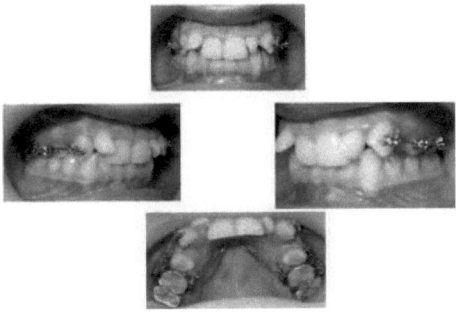

Partial arches

After 5 months we have closed the spaces left by extracted teeth and done the briquetting of all maxillary arches.

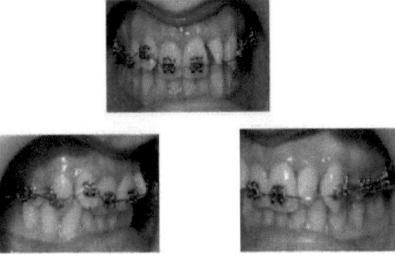

Briquetting of maxillary arch

After 9 months of maxillary teeth alignment, a device was placed in both inferior arches.

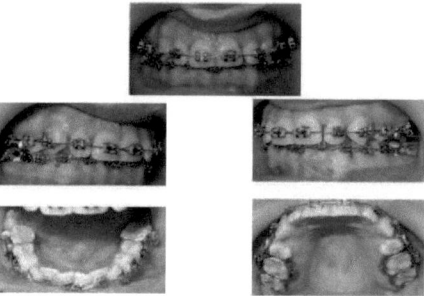

Briquetting of both arches

After 15 months of treatment alignment of both arches was achieved

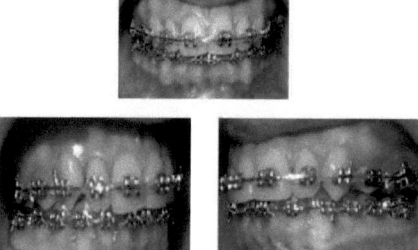

15 month treatment

While active treatment was completed after 18 months and intraoral images before and after treatment show the harmonious alignment of teeth in both arches. .

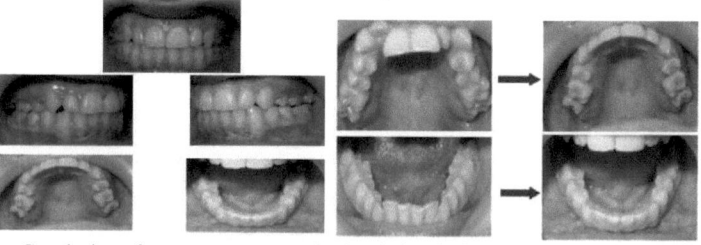

Conclusion of treatment   Occlusal view before and after treatment

Cephalometric data after the treatment show that skeletal values have not changed after treatment. So, we only managed to achieve dental disguise, without successfully affecting the skeletal base.

	Before	After treatment
• **SNA =**	*82°*	*81°*
• **SNB =**	*77°*	76°
• **ANB =**	5°	4°
• **WITS =**	3 mm	3 mm
• **GoGnSN =**	30°	31°
• **FM =**	22°	23°
• **MM =**	20°	22°
• <u>L</u> to A-Po =	6 mm	7 mm
• <u>L</u> to A-Po =	0 mm	1 mm
• <u>I</u> to Max Plane =	110 mm	106 mm
• I to Mand Plane =	93mm	96 mm

The patient informed us that she had sought orthodontic help before, but was told that she had to wait until all teeth had erupted in order to start treatment. If we were to determine the patient's biological age and observed that she was at the peak of growth, orthodontic work would be successful in skeletal level. Disadvantages of delayed treatment in this case were:

1. Not effects in the skeletal, orthopedic level
2. Convex profile not entirely corrected
3. Sacrificing 2 premolars
4. Costly therapy
5. Establishment of a permanent retainer in the maxilla and portable one in the lower arch for an indefinite amount of time to maintain the achieved results.

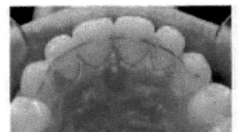 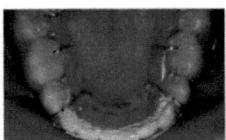

Retainer after treatment

3. Patient O.L. Anomaly: Class III dental and skeletal.

Patient history:

Patient (O. S.), 14 years and 11 months; Female was seeking treatment for a moderate dental and skeletal malocclusion of class III, the main concern was the negative anterior over-jet and a non-aesthetic smile. The patient profile was concave as occlusion and central relation. Clinical examination showed a facial type (appearance) of grade III, with competence strained lips. It was a prominent lower lip. Vertical facial proportions were normal without significant asymmetry. The first molars were extracted under (teeth 46 and 36).

45

Top right plant was endodontically treated years ago and was decolorized. Front teeth were abraded. Intraoral examination showed class III canine on the right side and I-st class on the left. It had negative over-jet 2.5 mm and overbite 2 mm. Oral hygiene was good.

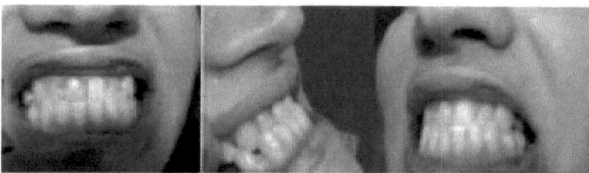

Intraoral view before treatment

Cephalometric evaluation (Figure 9-100) showed that maxilla was easily retrusive in relation to cranial base (SNA 78∘) and the mandible was at an advanced forward position at the cranial base (SNB 82∘). ANB (-4∘) showed a skeletal report of class III. Maxillary and mandibular incisors were easily proclined. Mandibular plane was normal at the cranial base (SN-Mego = 30∘). Cephalometric analysis showed a skeletal problem with prognathic mandibles and retarded maxillae.

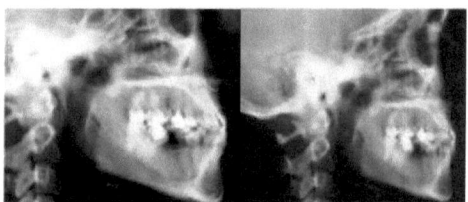

Cephalometric X-Ray before treatment

Data from anamnesis, with regard to the secondary sexual signs, showed that the girl had passed the stage of growth and skeletal development. Age determination by panoramic X-ray shows a dental age of over 16 years.

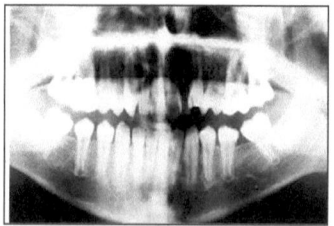

Panoramic X-Ray

The determination of skeletal age by examining the hand and wrist radiographs, indicate that the patient is in stage 9, so there is no potential for patient's further growth.

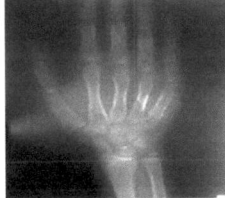

Hand and wrist X-ray

Based on the following data:
Chronological age: 14 years 11 months.
Skeletal age: 16 years 1 month.
Given that the patient has no growth potential, it was the intent of orthodontic treatment to correct dental grade and alignment of teeth in superior and inferior arcade. For this purpose, treatment objectives were:
1. Correction of anterior intersection;
2. The creation of the report of I-st dental class;
3. Proclination of upper front teeth;
4. Correction of overbite, over- jet and the median line;
5. Provision of an aesthetic smile.

To achieve these objectives a protocol of non-surgical treatment was decided.
The following treatment was implemented:
The removable maxillary device was applied, with Z springs and sagittal screw which was placed the 4 upper anterior teeth. The dental apparatus had a synthetic resin posterior surface for the disocclusion of anterior teeth. Patient was advised to wear the device for 24 hours, even during meals.

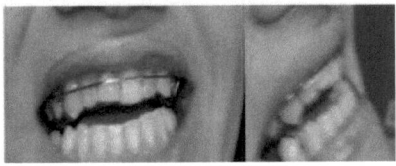

Portable device

Results of treatment:
The result was achieved in 16 months. The goals of treatment were achieved. I-st dental class ratio was achieved, with a positive over-jet and optimal overbite. Maxillary incisors were proclinated, resulting in better the prominence of the upper lip and better facial profile.

Second treatment: After the completion of active treatment, the upper front teeth were filled with composite in order to shape the eroded teeth. No retainer was placed after treatment. Orthodontic correction was only dento-alveolar, which was confirmed by cephalometric results before and after treatment and the superposition of cephalometric data before and after treatment

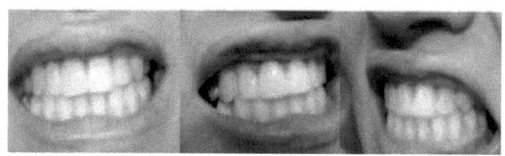

After orthodontic and aesthetic treatment

Values	Before	After	Difference
SNA	78+	78+	0+
SNB	82+	82+	0+
ANB	-4+	-4+	0+
1 max/Sna-Snp	108+	112+	4+
1 mand/Go Me	96+	94+	2+
Over-jet (mm)	-2.5	3	5.5
Overbite (mm)	2	4	2
SN/Me Go	30+	31+	1+

Cephalometric values before and after treatment

If the patient would have been treated in the period of growth, orthodontic work would be effective in skeletal level. Disadvantages of delayed treatment in this case were:
3. Aesthetic filling of the front teeth as a result of erosion of the anterior junction Veneers
4. Costly therapy

4. The patient E.D. Anomaly: III-d Class dental and skeletal.
Patient history: The patient (ED) 10 years and 8 months, female, had a case of moderate III-d class dental and skeletal malocclusion, the main concern was reverse anterior over-jet and a non- aesthetic smile. The patient's profile was concave in centric occlusion while in still position.

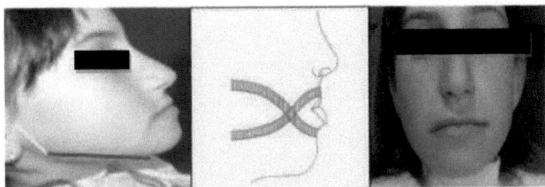
Extra-oral view before treatment

Intraoral examination showed class III canine and molar. Reverse over-jet was 3 mm and 4 mm overbite.

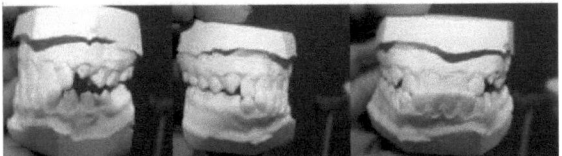
Intraoral view before treatment

The cephalometric evaluation showed a case of retrusive maxilla in the cranial base (SNA 77°) and the mandible was advanced in forward position in relation to the cranial base (SNB 83°). ANB (-6°) showed a class III skeletal ratio. Maxillary incisors had a normal ratio in connection with the cranial base and bi-spinal plane while mandibular incisors were slightly proclined. Mandibular plane was normal in relation to cranial base (SN-Mego = 29°). Cephalometric analysis showed a skeletal problem with prognathic mandible and retarded maxillae.

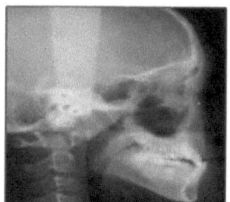

Cephalometric X-ray before treatment

The data from anamnesis with regard to secondary sexual signs showed that the girl was between I and II period of growth and development.

Age determination by dental panoramic X-ray shows a dental age of 10 years and 6 months.

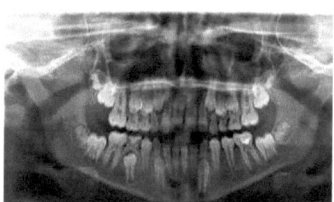

Panoramic X-ray

Whereas determination of skeletal age by the hand and wrist radiographs, indicates that the patient is in stage III, namely the patient has not yet entered the pubertal peak.

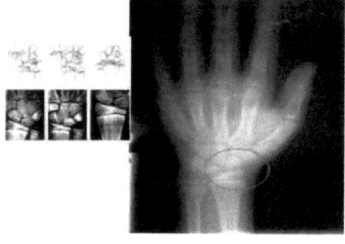 Hand X-ray

Given the following data:
Chronological age: 10 years 8 months.
Skeletal age: 10 years 6-8 months.

Because the patient has growing potential, the objective was orthodontic and orthopedic treatment to correct dental and skeletal problems.

A portable, functional apparatus was used; the twin-block device was placed in the upper and lower jaw. The dental apparatus had a synthetic resin posterior surface Apparatus had posterior surface with resin and posterior extension in the upper jaw and in the anterior mandible. Both surfaces join at a 70° angle that provokes an anterior advancement of the maxilla and prevents advancement of the mandible. A vestibular arc with an application of resin in its surface was placed on the lower proclinated anterior teeth. Patient was advised to wear the device for 24 hours, even during meals.

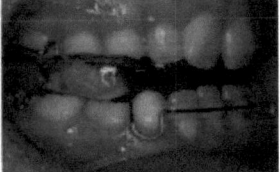

Twin-block 2 device

Results of treatment:
Treatment lasted 8 months. The goals of treatment were achieved. Facial profile was normal with a prominent upper lip.

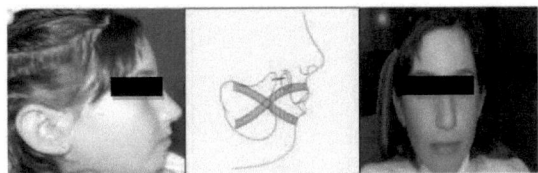

Extra-oral view after treatment

Class I dental and skeletal ratio was achieved, positive over-jet and optimal overbite was created. Orthodontic and orthopedic correction was not only in the dento- alveolar level, but also skeletal, confirmed by cephalometric values after treatment. Results were satisfactory because patient's growth potential was exploited in favor of modifying the skeletal structures.

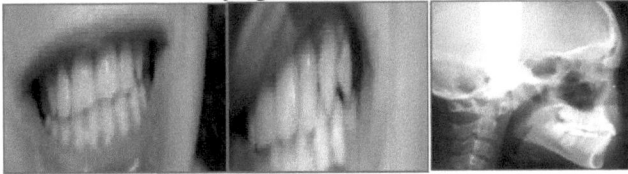

After orthodontic treatment   Cephalometric X-ray

5. Patient E.C. Anomaly: Skeletal open bite.

Patient history: The patient (EC) 9 years and 8 months, female, came to the clinic presenting as the main concern the anterior open bite and non- aesthetic gingival smile. Parents complained about the oral breathing of the girl. Intraoral examination showed the presence of bite open with anterior tongue thrust, compromised maxilla and maxillary anterior teeth malposition.

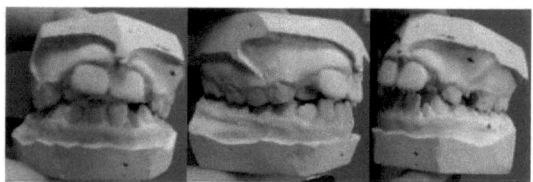

Intraoral view before orthodontic treatment

Cephalometric assessment of the maxilla and mandible showed almost normal ratios at the cranial base (SNA 80◦) (SNB 76◦). ANB (4◦) showed a skeletal report of class I with a tendency toward class II. Maxillary and mandibular incisive had a normal ratio in relation to the respective maxillary planes. All angles (between the mandibular planes to the cranial base, etc.) and ratio of facial features, showed the presence of skeletal open bite.

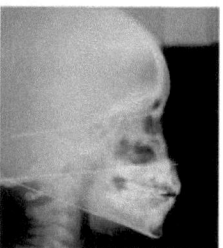

Cephalometric X-ray before treatment

The data from anamnesis with regard to the secondary sexual signs showed that the girl was between I and II period of growth and development.

Age determination by dental panoramic X-ray shows a dental age of over 16 years.

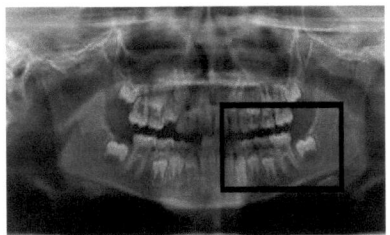

Panoramic X-ray

Whereas determination of skeletal age by the hand and wrist radiographs indicates that the patient is in the 2nd developmental stage, namely the patient has not yet entered the pubertal peak.

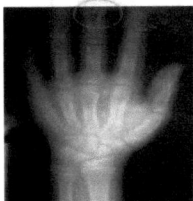

Hand and wrist X-ray

From the following data:
Chronological Age: 9 years 8 months.
Skeletal age: 10 years 1 month.

Given that the patient has growing potential, the goal was functional orthodontic treatment to correct skeletal problems.
Open bite as a result of posterior rotation of the mandible, is among the anomalies that must be addressed as early as possible.
Functional portable apparatus was placed in the upper jaw with an expanding screw; the posterior surface had a thick layer of synthetic resin for the for the purpose of intrusion in the process of alveolar posterior and consequently provoking anterior and upper rotation of the mandible. In the posterior portion was incorporated a "ball" of resin, which the patient was advised to touch with the tongue, to consciously eliminate the tongue thrust. Patient was advised to wear the device for 24 hours, even during meals.

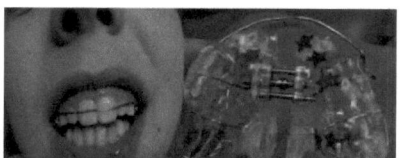

Functional apparatus

Results of treatment:
Treatment lasted for 11 months. The goals of treatment were achieved. It created optimum over-jet and overbite. Second treatment: After the end of active treatment, apparatus is kept as retainer at night only to maintain the results of the treatment until the end of growing cycle.

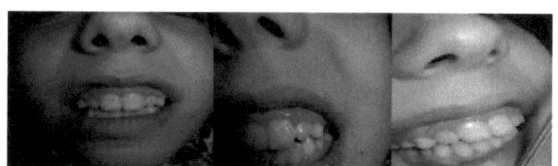

After orthodontic treatment

Orthodontic correction was not only dento-alveolar but also skeletal, confirmed by cephalometric values before and after treatment and the superposition of cephalometric data before and after treatment, where the vertical change of the open bite parameters is very visible..

Before treatment		After treatment	
FMIA	66	FMIA	68
FMA	24	FMA	24
IMPA	90	IMPA	88
SNA	80	SNA	79
SNB	76	SNB	76
ANB	4	ANB	3
AO BO	3mm	AO BO	2mm
PFH	45mm	PFH	46mm
AFH	66mm	AFH	68mm
INDEX	.68	INDEX	.67

Cephalometric values before and after treatment

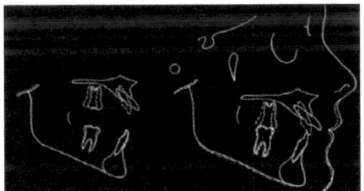

Cephalometric superimposing before and after treatment

6. Patient V.M. Anomaly: Class II/ dental and skeletal anomaly.

Patient is 11 years 6 months, came to the clinic for treatment of upper teeth, which burst out of lips. Extra-oral examination shows a convex profile, folded lips and interposition of the lower lip. 1/3 inferior dimensions.

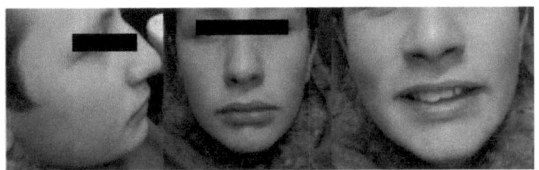

Extra-oral view

Intraoral View indicates the presence of over-jet 12 mm, dental grade II and presence of a deep traumatic bite.

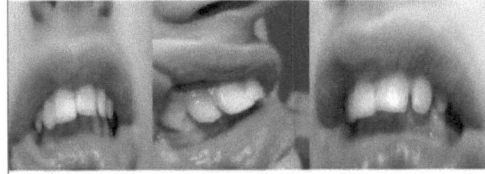

Intraoral view

Deciphering of cephalometric values highlights grade II dental and skeletal anomaly.

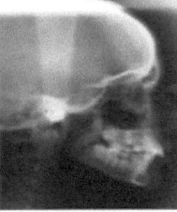

Cephalometric X-ray

Given the chronological age of the patient we could delay functional treatment for several months. Whereas according to secondary sexual characteristics the boy has not yet reached a maximum maturity phase (pubertal peak), but it was close to this stage. Dental age showed that the patient was 12 years and 4 months, and skeletal age was in stage 4, or 12 years and 8 months.

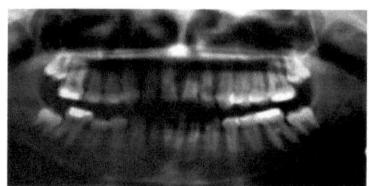

Panoramic X-ray

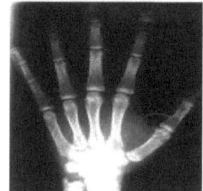

Hand and wrist X-ray

Given the following data:
Chronological age: 11 years 6 months.
Skeletal age: 12 years 4-8 months.
Malocclusion: Class II / 1.
We decided to begin with functional orthopedic treatment immediately. An activator was applied for the anterior advancement of mandible and the maxillary and dental retrusion.

The apparatus was equipped with lip-plumber to model labial and mental muscles, to help the anterior mandible advancement.

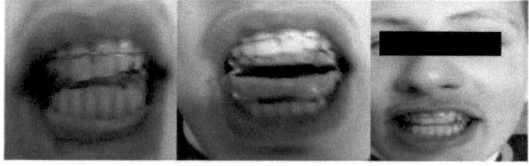

Functional apparatus

After 1 year of active use, the apparatus was kept for another year at night to maintain the achieved results. As shown in extra-oral view, the patient has signs of visible vegetation in the face, one of the indicators that the boy has entered the stage of pubertal growth.

Completion of successful treatment resulted in class I of dental and skeletal stage. Cephalometric reports after treatment show normal skeletal bases of the sagittal and vertical planes.

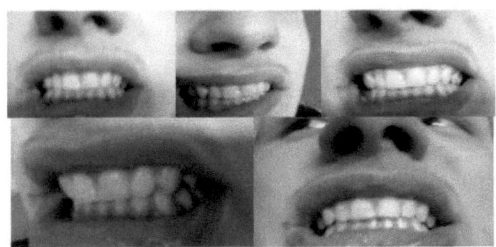

After treatment

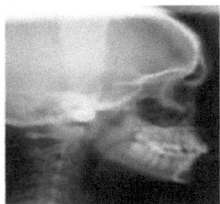

Cephalometric X-ray after treatment

7. DISCUSSION

With regard to patients with skeletal abnormalities and the time treatment starts, by applying Chi-Square test, a statistically significant difference was found between groups (by time of onset of treatment) in relation to treatment results.

• In the group that was treated *at pubertal peak*, results were satisfactory in 70% of cases much higher than those of the other group which was treated after pubertal peak which was (30%) and the group treated before the pubertal peak (30%) (p = 0.019). This indicates that if patients are treated during their pubertal peak we have better treatment results.

• Patients treated *before pubertal peak* (40) where:

• 12 (30%) patients received timely and successful treatment, and the end result was that 2 (16.7%) patients had discrepancies, and in 10 (83.3%) patients there was compliance between chronological and biological age.

• 14 (35%) patients treatment lasted more than 2 years, and the end result was that 10 (71.4%) patients had discrepancies and in 4 (28.6%) patients there was compliance between chronological and biological age.

• 14 (35%) patients treatment was done in 2 stages, and the end result was that 11 (78.6%) patients had discrepancies and in 3 (21.4%) patients there was compliance between chronological and biological age.

• Patients treated *during pubertal peak* (40) where:

• 28 (70%) patients had satisfactory outcome, and the end result was that 10 (35.7%) patients had discrepancies and in 18 (64.3%) patients there was compliance between chronological and biological age

• 12 (30%) patients had extended treatment, and the end result was that 6 (50.0%) patients had discrepancies and in 6 (50.0%) patients there was compliance between chronological and biological age.

• Patients treated *after pubertal peak* where:

• 9 (22.5%) patients had unsatisfactory results, end result was:

• 2 (22.2%) patients had discrepancies and in 7 (77.8%) patients there was compliance between chronological and biological age.

• 19 (47.5%) patients had an extension in the duration of their treatment, and the end result was:

10 (52.6%) patients had discrepancies and in 9 (47.4%) patients there was compliance between chronological and biological age.

• 12 (30%) patients had satisfactory results, and the end result was:

3 (25.0%) patients had discrepancies and in 9 (75.0%) patients there was compliance between chronological and biological age.

8. CONCLUSIONS

About 2/3 of orthodontic patients have malocclusion, where growth and development play an important role in the success or failure of treatment and directly affect the decision on the use of extra-oral mechanisms, functional apparatus, extractions or orthognathic surgery.

Orthodontists must understand events associated with growth and development because the maturity stages have a decisive role in diagnosis, treatment planning and extension of treatment, as well as the prognosis of malocclusion. Therefore determination of the type of growth for each individual patient is a fundamental factor in the success of orthodontic treatment.

Growth and development should be considered as a kind of energy. Why should this energy be used with caution? The answer to this question will clarify the timing of orthopedic treatment, which includes guiding the development of dento-alveolar and skeletal structures. Preventing undesirable changes associated with growth and using to our advantage the desirable effects of growth, constitutes the general principle of orthopedic treatment. In orthodontics and dento-facial orthopedics, skeletal maturity status in a growing patient influences the selection and application of orthodontic treatment procedures. Favorable orthopedic effects for patients with skeletal problems occur only when treatment begins during the optimal maturing stage. Meanwhile, it is recommended that the best time for surgical correction of skeletal problems is after completion of growth. Considerable variations in development exist between individuals of the same chronological age; this led to the concept of evaluating the biological or physiological maturity.

Given that the definition of secondary sexual characteristics requires a longitudinal study and a compilation of an anamnesis in close cooperation with parents (especially the mother, which is not always possible), we cannot consider this biological indicator as a major determinant in defining biological age, but as an extra help in our "screening".

In defining dental maturity Demirian system is most widely used, but we have referred to other systems such as the Nordic ones (38). According to various authors quoted above, dental age determination is made based on the stages of dental mineralization (53). Growth and calcification of dental tissue was used to determine the dental age. Calcification of teeth is more accurate than teeth eruption, because the time of eruption of a tooth is very difficult to determine, and calcification is an ongoing process that can be estimated by keeping permanent records such as panoramic X-ray, and therefore should be considered as a better tool for evaluating physiological maturity (50).

X-ray of the hand and wrist is one of the most popular biological indicators used by orthodontists to assess skeletal development. It is reported that there is a close relation between bone maturity of hand and facial growth.

Descriptive statistics were calculated for subjects in each age group (7-15 years).

1. Comparison of differences between the chronological, dental and skeletal age resulted in substantial discrepancies 63.1%. Correlates test was used for comparison and find the connection between the respective maturing stages of the hand and dental maturation.

2. Comparison of differences between the chronological, dental and skeletal age was conducted in both sexes. Sexual dimorphism exists in each stage of skeletal maturity. The average age of the subjects was generally younger in women than in men. So, women are 2.6 times more likely than men to reach an earlier biological mature age. Likewise, early maturity is more prevalent among women than among boys and there is possibility of the influence of hormonal factors.

3. The lower values of the average difference was seen in younger age groups (6-9 years), while significant differences between the estimated age and the chronological age were seen in both sexes in the older age group (9 -12 years).

4. As our research concluded (but also is completely certified by contemporary foreign literature), the most secure, the most reliable method for determining the stages of growth and development of a child, is the determination of skeletal age by radiography of the hand and the determination of dental age not based on eruption stages (as has been done so far), but by observing the calcification stages of permanent teeth. However, skeletal age is the method mostly used compared with dental age, due to the lack of the age limit.

5. Skeletal problems in any kind of orientation plane (sagittal, transversal, vertical) should be treated at the end of stage 3 (when the evident ossification of the pisiform bone has occurred, it is the start of the uncinate bone ossification and the epiphysis and diaphysis of radius have equal width), and the beginning of stage 4 (when the primary mineralization of the sesamoid bone is present and we have the complete ossification of the uncinate bone, therefore the stage corresponding to the pubertal growth spurt). So it is a fact of great clinical importance that the orthodontic treatment options have a defined individual timing for different patients. Not all children should start orthopedic treatment at age 11; today age is defined by 2 very powerful indicators.

Use of chronological age alone increases the possibility of clinical errors, which in a second stage would affect not only the results of the treatment, but also its extension in time, if there are no permanent results or to put it differently the result will be failure and an increase of costs and time, not only for the patient but also the doctor. Evaluation and determination of intense growth periods that occur during human maturity provides important clinical information for orthodontic, orthopedic treatment and retentive procedures.

Based on the level of skeletal maturity doctors determine the type of treatment to be applied (orthodontic, orthopedic or surgical).

9. RECOMMENDATIONS

Based on our study and foreign literature we concluded that chronological age is a poor indicator in the determination of skeletal growth. Usage of the chronological age alone will increase chances of clinical error, adversely affecting the outcome of treatment and have a negative impact on the patient. In order to achieve success in the use of chosen mechanotherapy and prognosis of the future treatment of skeletal abnormalities of the class II, class III, open bite, cross bite, this process should be preceded by the accurate determination of biological age.

- Skeletal maturity is to be determined by referring to radiographic seeming calcified structures of the hand and wrist, since it is the most reliable and safer method.
- It is important to point out that not only orthodontists, but also maxillofacial surgeons before performing an orthognathic surgery should determine the skeletal age. Surgical corrections in these patients should be done after completion of growth.
- Orthodontic treatment options have defined individual timing for each individual patient. Not taking into consideration the exact age of the patient means failure of the result achieved or prolongation of treatment in the final stage.

Nowadays medicine requires constant vigilance, dynamic, professional check-ups for every doctor who works with children who are growing. *There is nothing more beautiful than to use these positive features for the good of the patients.*

10. BIBLIOGRAPHY

1- G. Koch.S. Poulsen. Pediatric dentistry.2001.47-52. Crescita e svilupo post-natali.

2- Zerin JM, Hernandez RJ. Hand Clin. 1991 Feb;7(1):53-62. Approach to skeletal maturation. Department of Radiology, University of Michigan Hospitals, Ann Arbor.

3-Cox LA. Acta Paediatr Suppl. 1997 Nov;423:107-8. The biology of bone maturation and ageing.

4-Soegiharto BM, Cunningham SJ, Moles DR. Am J Orthod Dentofacial Orthop. 2008 Aug;134(2):217 Skeletal maturation in Indonesian and white children assessed with hand-wrist and cervical vertebrae methods.

5- Smith RJ.Am J Orthod. 1980 Jan;77(1):75-8. Misuse of hand-wrist radiographs.

6- Sahin Sağlam AM, Gazilerli U. J Orofac Orthop. 2002 Nov;63(6):454-62.The relationship between dental and skeletal maturity.

7- Freitas D, Maia J, Beunen G, Lefevre J, Claessens A, Marques A, Rodrigues A, Silva C, Crespo M, Thomis M, Sousa A, Malina R. Ann Hum Biol. 2004 Jul-Aug;31(4):408-20. Skeletal maturity and socioeconomic status in Portuguese children and youths: the Madeira growth study.

8- Akridge M, Hilgers KK, Silveira AM, Scarfe W, Scheetz JP, Kinane DF. Am J Orthod Dentofacial Orthop. 2007 Aug;132(2):185-90. Childhood obesity and skeletal maturation assessed with Fishman's hand-wrist analysis.

9- Kimura K. Am J Phys Anthropol. 1983 Apr;60(4):491-7. Skeletal maturity and bone growth in twins.

10- Coutinho S, Buschang PH, Miranda F. Am J Orthod Dentofacial Orthop. 1993 Sep;104(3):262-8. Relationships between mandibular canine calcification stages and skeletal maturity.

11- Serinelli S, Panetta V, Pasqualetti P, Marchetti D. Leg Med (Tokyo). 2011 May;13(3):120-33. Epub 2011 Mar 4. Accuracy of three age determination X-ray methods on the left hand-wrist: a systematic review and meta-analysis.

12- Mauchamp OP, Nanda SK..Rev Orthop Dento Faciale. 1975 Jan;9(1):47-72.[Prediction of the amount of growth as a function of the biological age].

13- Al Khal HA, Wong RW, Rabie AB. Skeletal Radiol. 2008 Mar;37(3):195-200. Epub 2007 Oct 3.Elimination of hand-wrist radiographs for maturity assessment in children needing orthodontic therapy.

14- Gilli G.Horm Res. 1996;45 Suppl 2:49-52.The assessment of skeletal maturation.

15- Kucukkeles N, Acar A, Biren S, Arun T. J Clin Pediatr Dent. 1999 Fall;24(1): 47- 52. Comparisons between cervical vertebrae and hand-wrist maturation for the assessment of skeletal maturity.

16- Houston WJ.Eur J Orthod. 1980;2(2):81-93. Relationships between skeletal maturity estimated from hand-wrist radiographs and the timing of the adolescent growth spurt.

17- Grave K, Townsend G. Aust Orthod J. 2003 Nov;19(2):33-45.Hand-wrist and cervical vertebral maturation indicators: how can these events be used to time Class II treatments?

18- Uysal T, Ramoglu SI, Basciftci FA, Sari Z. Am J Orthod Dentofacial Orthop. 2006 Nov;130(5):622-8. Chronologic age and skeletal maturation of the cervical vertebrae and hand-wrist: is there a relationship?

19- Stiehl J, Müller B, Dibbets J. J Orofac Orthop. 2009 Jul;70(4):327-35. Epub 2009 Aug 2. The development of the cervical vertebrae as an indicator of skeletal maturity: comparison with the classic method of hand-wrist radiograph.

20- Lai EH, Liu JP, Chang JZ, Tsai SJ, Yao CC, Chen MH, Chen YJ, Lin CP.J Formos Med Assoc. 2008 Apr;107(4):316-25. Radiographic assessment of skeletal maturation stages for orthodontic patients: hand-wrist bones or cervical vertebrae?

21- Acta Anat (Basel). 1996;155(3):206-11. Skeletal maturation of wrist and hand ossification centers in normal Spanish boys and girls: a study using the Greulich-Pyle method.

22- Jiménez-Castellanos J, Carmona A, Catalina-Herrera CJ, Viñuales M. Indian J Dent Res. 2011 Mar-Apr;22(2):309-16. Evaluation of skeletal maturation by comparing the hand wrist radiograph and cervical vertebrae as seen in lateral cephalogram.

23-Björk A. Trans Eur Orthod Soc. 1972:61-74. Timing of interceptive orthodontic measures based on stages of maturation.

24- S.Barnasconi,L.Iughetti, L. Ghizzoni. In "Endocrinologia Pediatrica'. McGraw-Hill 2000

25-Preston Sh.1976.Modelli di mortallita nelle popolazioni nazionali :con particulare riferimento alle cause di morte registrate.NeëYork:Academic Press.

26-Mul D, Fredriks AM, van Buuren S, Oostdijk W, Verllove –Vanhorick SP, et al. 2001, Lo svilupo puberale nei Paesi Bassi 1965-1997, Pediatr Res 50. 479-486.

27-Cole TJ, 2003, La tendenza secolare di crescita umana fisica: Una vista biologic.Hum Biol Econ 1: 161-168.

28- Modello di crescita fisica e sessuale dei bambini indiani benestanti 5-18 anni di eta. Indiano Pediatr 1992,29:940-949.

29- Graham MJ.Larsen U.Xu X. Trend secolare di eta al menarca in Cina: Un caso di studio di due contee rurali nella provinca di Anhiu.J Biosoc Sci 1999, 31:257- 267.

30-Floud R, Ëacher K, Gregory A. 1990, Altezza,la salute e la storia :lo stato nutrizionale nel Regno Unito,1970-1980.Cambridge studi di popolazione, economia e societa nel tempo passato. Cambridge University Press.

31- Grumbch MM. Styne DM.Puberta: Ontogenesi ,neuroendocrinologia, fisiologia e disturbi In:JD Wilson, Foster DW, HM Kronenberg, PR Larsen,eds Williams Textbook di Endocrinologia . ed. Philadelphia :WB Saunders Co, 1998,p. 1509-1625.

32- Wyshak G, Frisch RE.L'evidenca di un trend secolare di eta del menarca. N Engl J med 1982.306:1033-1035.

33- Frich RE, Revelle Altezza R. Peso al menarcha e l'ipotesi di peso corporeo critico ed eventi adolescente.Scienza 1970, 169: 397-399.

34- Larsen P. timing affetivo e pravalenza di sovrapeso nelle ragazze adolescenti degli Stati Uniti. Am J sanita publica 2001 ,91: 642-644.

35-Tahirove HF .Eta menarca e lo stress della guerra.un esempio dalla Bosnia.Eur J Pediatr 1998,157:978-980.

36- Preberg Z, Bralic ,Modifiche I. in eta menarca nelle bambine esposte a condizioni di guerra. Am J Hum Biol 2000,12: 503-508.

37- Adolfsson S, Westphal O. svilupo puberale precoce nelle bambine adottate da paesi dell'Estremo Oriente. Pediatr Res 1981, 15:82.

38- Kataja M, Nystrom M, Aine L,Dental maturity standarts in southern Finland.Proc Finn Dent Soc 1989,187-97.

39- Hanlon PM, Radiographic considerations in pedodontics. J Pedod 1985,9; 285-301.

40- Demirijan A.buschang PH ,Tanguay R, Patterson DK, Interrelationships among measures of somatic ,skeletal,dental,and sexual maturity.

41- Hagg U ,Taranger J. Dental development ,dental age and tooth counts. Angle Orthodontists.

42- Lervik T.Cowley G. Dental radiographic screening in children. J.Dent Child 1983; 50: 128-135.

43- Bodzsar EB. 2000.Studi sulla maturazione sessuale dei bambini ungheresi .Szegediensis Acta Biologica 44: 155-165.

44-Daw SF. Eta della puberta i ragazzi a Lipsia,1727-49, come indicato dalla voce rotta nei membri di JS Bach coro. 1970. Hum. Biol. 42. 87-89.

45- Statistics Norway. Annuario statistico dela Norvegia.2005. Statistics Norway. 7 p.

46-Stearns SC. 1992. L'evoluzione delle storie di vita .New York:Oxford.

47- University of California ,Berkeley USA, e Max Planx Institute per la ricerca demografica(Germania). La mortalita database umano.

48- Frisch RE. 2006. Prevenzione dell'HIV in adolescenti. Science 311; 337.

49- Bjork A.Timing of interceptive orthodontic measures based on stages of maturation. Trans Eur Orthod Soc 1972;45:61-74.

50- Demirjian A. Dentition. In:FalknerF,Tanner JM,eds.Human growth.London Bailliere Tindall,1982.

51- Greulich W, Pyle SI. Radiographic atlas of skeletal development of the hand and wrist. California: Stanford University Press,1959.

52- Tanner JM,whitehouse RH,Marshall WA,Healy MJR ,Goldstein H. Assessment of skeletal maturity and prediction of adult height (TW2 method). London: Academic Press ,1975.

53- Human Development Reports ,United Nations Development Programme,2004.

54- Hagg U,: The pubertal growth spurt and maturity indicators of dental, skeletal and pubertal development. A prospective longitudinal study of Swedish urban children. Thesis, Malmo. Sweden 1980.

55- Hagg U, Taranger J, : Menarche and voice change as indicators of the pubertal growth spurt, Acta Odontol, Scand,38:179-186,1980.

56- Hagg U, Taranger J,: Skeletal stages of the hand and wrist as indicators of pubertal growth spurt. Acta Odontol, Scand,38; 187-200.1980.

57-Healy M.J.R: Statistics of growth standarts. In Falkner,F,and Tanner J.M: Human growth, London. Demirjian A, Buschang PH, Tanguay R, Patterson DK. Interrelationships among measures of somatic,skeletal,dental and sexual maturity.Am J Orthod 1985 Nov;88(5):433-8.

58-Flores-Mir C, Mauricio FR, Orellana MF, Major PË, Association between growth stunting with dental development and skeletal maturation stage. Angle Orthod 2005 Nov;75(6):935-40.

59-Hagg U, Taranger J. Dental development,dentale age and tooth counts. Angle Orthod 1985 Apr;55(2),93-107.

60-Heuze Y, Chabadel O, Braga J, Bley D. The impact of socioeconomic status on the estimation of non-adult dental age.Orthod Fr 2005;76(4),309-16.

61-Kromeyer K, Hauspie RC, Susanne C.Socioeconomic factors and growth during childhood and early adolescence in Jena children Ann Hum Biol 1997 Jul-Aug;24(4):343-53.

62-Kromeyer K, Wurschi F. Correlation between physical development and dentition based on the Jena Longitudinal Study.Anthropol Anz 1996 Sep;54(3):255-66.

63-Maber M, Liversidge HM, Hector MP.Accuracy of age estimation of radiographic methods using developing teeth.Forensic Sci Int 2006 May;15(1):68-73.Epub 2006 Mar 14

64-Smiech-Slomkoska G, Jarnecka B, Physical development and teeth ageof children aged 7-10 lat. Czas Stomatol 1990 Jul;43(7):434-8.

65-Benso L, Vannelli S, Pastorian L, Angius P, Milani S. Main problems associated with bone age and maturity evaluation.Bone Maturat 1996;2:42-48.

66-Bjork A. Timing of interceptive orthodontic measures based on stages of maturation.Trans Europ Orthod Soc 1972;61.

67-Carpenter CT, Lester EL. Skeletal age determination in young children:analysis of the regions of the hand-wrist film. J Pediatr Orthop 1993;13(1):76-79.

68-Franchi L, Baccetti T, McNamara JA Jr. Mandibular growth as related to cervical vertebral maturation and body height.Am J Orthod Dentofacial Orthop 2000;118:335-340

69-Garn SM, Rohmann GE. Variability in order of ossification of bony centers of the hand-wrist.Am J Phys Anthropol 1960; 18:219-230.

70-Groell R, Lindbichler F, Riepl T. The reliability of bone age determination in central European children using the GP method. Br J Radiol 1999;72:461-464

71-Hassel B, Farman A. Skeletal maturation evaluation using cervical vertebrae.Am J Orthod Dentofacial Orthop 1995;107:58-66.

72-Hellsing E. Cervical vertebral dimensions in 8-,11-,and 15-year-old children.Acta Odontol Scand 1991;49:207-213.

73-Lambarski D. Skeletal age assessment utilizing cervical vertebrae.Thesis,University of Pittsburgh, Pennsylvania;1972.

74-Mora S, Boechat I, Pietka E, Huang HK, Gilsanz V. Skeletal age determinations in children of European and African Descent:Applicability of the Greulich and Pyle Standards. Pediatr Res 2001;50:624-628.

75-So LL. Skeletal maturation of the hand and wrist and its correlation with dental development.Aust Orthod J 1997; 15:1-9.

76-So LL. Correlation of sexual maturation with skeletal age of southern Chinese girls.Aust Orthod J 1997; 4:215-217.

77-Bowden BD. Epiphyseal changes in the hand/wrist area as indicator of adolescent stage.Aust Orthod J 1976;4:87-104.

78-Brown T, Barrett MJ, Grave KC. Facial growth and skeletal maturation at adolescence.Danish Dent 1971;75:1211-1222.

79-Chapman S. Ossification of the adductor sesamoid and the adolescent growth spurt.Angle Orthod 1972;42:236-244.

80-Fishman LS. Radiographic evaluation of skeletal maturation.A clinically oriented method based on hand-wrist films.Angle Orthod 1982;52:88-112.

81-Gandini P, Manchini M, Andreani F. A comparison of hand wrist bone and cervical vertebral analyses in measuring skeletal maturation.Angel Orthod 2006;76(6):984-9.

82-Grave KC, Brown T. Skeletal ossification and the adolescent growth spurt.Am J Orthod 1976;6:611-619.

83-Hagg U, Taranger J. Maturation indicators and the pubertal growth spurt.Am J Orthod 1982;88:299-309.

84-Hassel B, Farman A. Skeletal maturation evaluation using cervical vertebrae.Am J Orthod Dentofacial Orthop 1995;107:58-66.

85-Alkhal HA, Wong RWK, Rabie ABM. Correlation between Chronological Age,Cervical Vertebral Maturation and Fishman's Skeletal Maturity Indicators in Southerm Chinese.Angel Orthod 2008;78(4):591-6.

86-Heligman L. Pollard, 1980.Il modello al'eta di mortalita. Jour Artuari Inst 107: 49-75

87- Preston Sh. 1976.Modelli di mortalita nelle popolazioni :con particolare riferimento alle cause di morte registrate.New York,Academic Press.

88- Cambell B. Mbizo M. 2006.Maturazione riptoduttiva ,la crescita somatica e il testosterone tra i ragazzi dello Zimbabwe. Ann Hum Biol 33. 17-25.

89- Argawal DK. Argawal NK. Modello di crescita fisica e sessuale dei bambini indiani bnestanti 5-18 anni di eta .Indiano Pediatr. 1992, 29: 240-949

90- Adair LS. Gordon – Larsen P. Timing affetivo e prevalenca di sovrepesso nelle ragazze adolescenti degli SU. Am J sanita publica 2001. 91: 642 – 644.

91-Cox LA. Am J Orthod Dentofacial Orthp.2008 Aug,134(2): 217-26"Skeletal maturation in Indonesian and white children assesed ëith hand –wrist and cervical vertebrae methods.

92-Koc A, Karaoglanoglu M, Erdogan M, Kosecik M, Cesur Y. Assessment of bone ages: is the Grulich-Pyle method sufficient for Turkish boys. Pediatr Int. 2001;43:662–665.

93- Buyukgebiz A, Eroglu Y, Karaman O, Kinik E. Height and weight measurements of male Turkish adolescents according to biological maturation. Acta Pediatr Jpn. 1994;36:80–83.

94- Silverman FN. In: Silverman FN, Jerald PK, eds. Caffey's Pediatric X-Ray Diagnosis: An Integrated Imaging Approach. St Louis, Mo: Mosby; 1993:1465–1529.

95-. Satoh M, Tanaka T, Hibi I. Analysis of bone age maturation and growth velocity in isolated growth hormone deficient boys with and without gonadal suppression treatment and in GH deficient boys with associated gonadotropin deficiency. J Pediatr Endocrinol Metab. 1997;10:615–622.

97. Ruf S, Pancherz H. Frontal sinus development as an indicator for somatic maturity at puberty. Am J Orthod Dentofacial Orthop.1996;110:476–482.

98.- Bjork A, Helm S. Prediction of the age of maximum pubertal growth in body height. Angle Orthod. 1967;37:134–143.

99.- Bergersen EO. The male adolescent facial growth spurt: its prediction and relation to skeletal maturation. Angle Orthod. 1972;42:319–338.

100-. Hagg U, Taranger J. Skeletal stages of the hand and wrist as indicators of the pubertal growth spun. Acta Odontol Scand. 1980;38:187–200.

101.- Krailassiri S, Anuwongnukroh N, Dechkunakorn S. Relationship between dental calcification stages and skeletal maturity indicators in Thai individuals. Angle Orthod. 2002;72:155–166.

102. Coutinho S, Buschang PH, Miranda F. Relationship between mandibular canine calcification stages and skeletal maturity. Am J Orthod Dentofacial Orthop. 1993;104:262–268.

103- Houston, W. J. Relationships between skeletal maturity estimated from hand-wrist radiographs and the timing of the adolescent growth spurt. Eur J Orthod 1980. 2:81–93.

104- Bowden, B. D. Sesamoid bone appearance as an indicator of adolescence. Aust Orthod J 1971. 2:242–248.

105- Lima JEO. Um plano de prevenção para consultório odontopediátrico. Rev Gaúcha Odontol. 1992;40(6):395-9.

106- Dowd FJ. Saliva and dental caries. Dent Clin North Am. 1999;43(4):579-97.

107- Fejerskov O, Nyvad B, Kidd EAM. Características clínicas e histológicas da cárie dentária. In: Fejerskov O, Kidd EAM. Cárie Dentária: a doença e seu tratamento clínico. São Paulo: Santos; 2005. p. 72-96.

108- Baker OD. Posteruptive changes in dental enamel. J Dent Res. 1966;45(Suppl 3):503-11. 109- Karen Elliot, Baby Bottles Can Cause Tooth Decay, Regional Specialist, Nutrition and Health Education,JacksonCounty,Missouri.

110- Bresolin, Shapiro E.T. Mouth Breathing Children: It's Relationship to Dentofacial Development . Al. American Journal of Orthodontics 1983.

111- Egil P. Harvold, DDS Ph.D.,L.L.D.Brittta S. Tamer, DDS, Kevin Varervik, DDS., and George Chierici, DDS "Facial appearance and dental occlusion in mpouth breathing" - American Journal of Orthodontics Vol 79. No. 4 April, 1981.

112- Donald G. Woodside, Sten Linder-Aronson, Anders Lundstrom, John William. American. "Mouth breathing with greater mandibular growth". Journal of Orthodontics July 1991.

113- Cheraskin E. and Ringdorf W. : Biology of the orthodontic patient:Relationship of chronolgic and dental age in terms of vitamin C state . Am . J . Ortho . : Jan 1972 , Vol . 42 No.1. 114- Malagola C, Caigiuri F.M ., Barrato E: Evaluation of dental age using qualitative radiographic analysis mondo- ortho.

115- Jaeger U : Dental age in dependence on the stage of selected physi ological development parameters - stomat 1990 Dec . 40 (12) : 511-514.

116- Carvalho A.A. Decarvalho A: Radiographic study of the development of permanent dentition of Brazilian children with chronologic age of 84 and 131 months. Odontol. Revy. 1991; 19 (1) : 31-39.

117- Leonard Rothenberg: Assessment of physical maturation and somatomedin levels during puberty. Am. J. Orth. 1977, 667-675.

118- Seymour Chertkow : Tooth mineralization as an indicator of the pubertal growth. AJO 1980, 79-81.

119- Leitte and co: Skeletal age assessment using fingers of the hand. AJO 1987, 492-498.

120- Fishman LS. Radiographic evaluation of skeletal maturation. A clinically oriented method based on hand-wrist films. Angle Orthod 1982;52:88-112.

121- Grave KC, Brown T. Skeletal ossification and the adolescent growth spurt. Am J Orthod 1982;82:299-309.

122-Davidson LE, Rodd lID. Interrelationship between dental age and chronological age in Somali children. Community Dent Health 2001;18:27–30. [From the Department of Child Dental Health, University of Sheffield, UK]

123-GALIĆ I, AMBARKOVA V, VODANOVIĆ , BRKIĆ H.Dental age calculation by Demirjian's method on children in Macedonia

124- Bastardo Ruby; Figuera Adriana; Rueda Yulmaira; Ortiz Mónica; Quirós Oscar; Farías Margarita ;Alcedo Carolina; Bastardo Ruby; Dorathys Fuenmayor; Godoy Sol; De Jurisic Aura; MazzaPatricia

Correlación entre edad cronológica y edad ósea - edad dental en pacientes del Diplomado de Ortodoncia Interceptiva,UGMA-2007
125- Karen Oerter Klein, Kimberly A. Larmore, Elizabeth de Lancey, Jaquelyn M. Brown, Robert V. Effect of Obesity on Estradiol Level, and Its Relationship to Leptin, Bone Maturation, and Bone Mineral Density in Children A. I. duPont Hospital for Children, Wilmington, Delaware 19899; and Indiana University Medical School, Indianapolis, Indiana 46206.

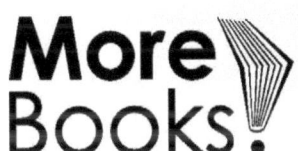

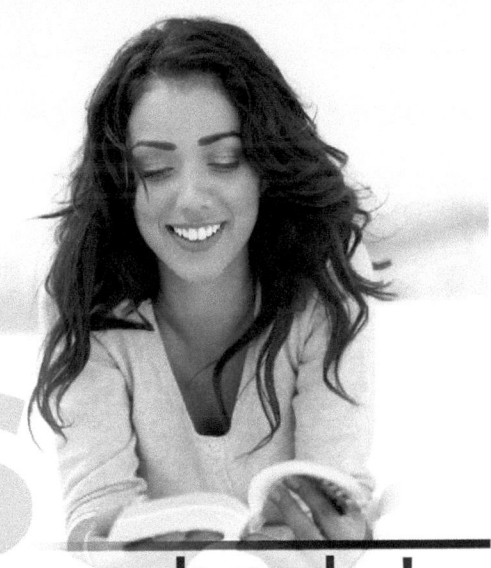

I want morebooks!

Buy your books fast and straightforward online - at one of the world's fastest growing online book stores! Environmentally sound due to Print-on-Demand technologies.

Buy your books online at
www.get-morebooks.com

Kaufen Sie Ihre Bücher schnell und unkompliziert online – auf einer der am schnellsten wachsenden Buchhandelsplattformen weltweit! Dank Print-On-Demand umwelt- und ressourcenschonend produziert.

Bücher schneller online kaufen
www.morebooks.de

OmniScriptum Marketing DEU GmbH
Heinrich-Böcking-Str. 6-8
D - 66121 Saarbrücken
Telefax: +49 681 93 81 567-9

info@omniscriptum.com
www.omniscriptum.com

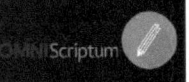

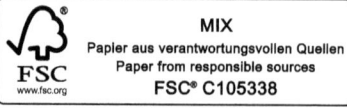

MIX
Papier aus verantwortungsvollen Quellen
Paper from responsible sources
FSC® C105338

Printed by Books on Demand GmbH, Norderstedt / Germany